5-INGREDIENT
FAMILY COOKBOOK

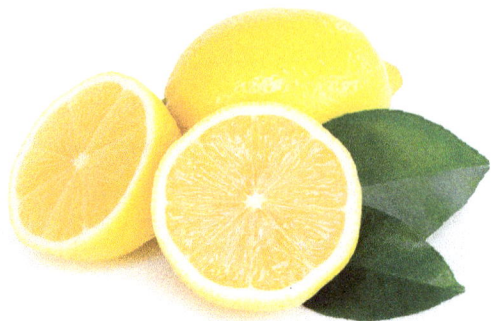

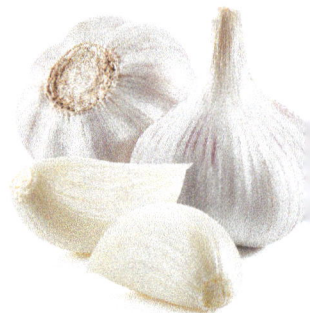

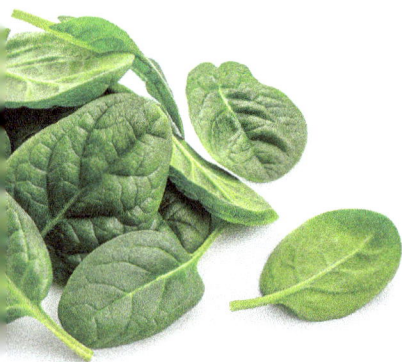

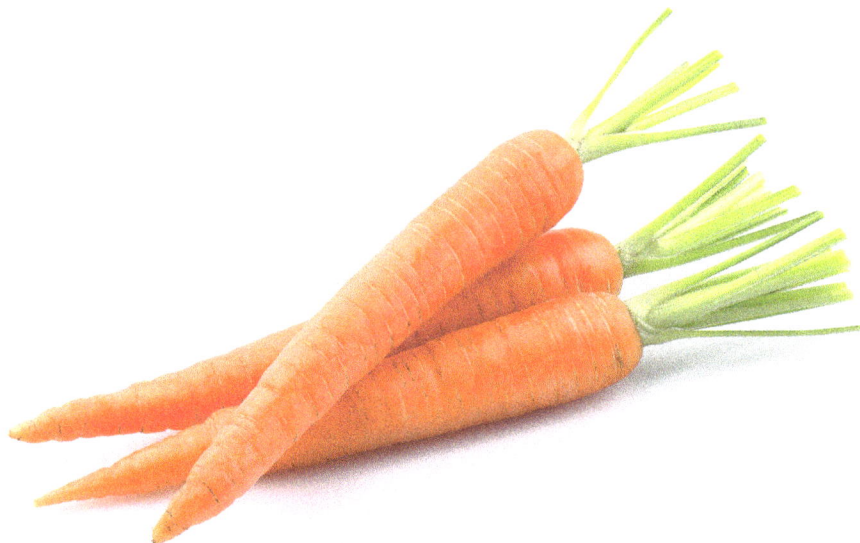

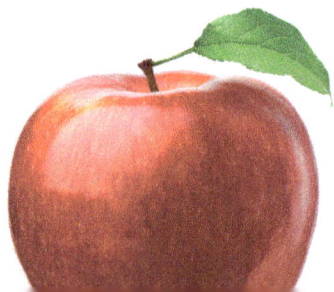

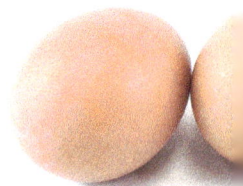

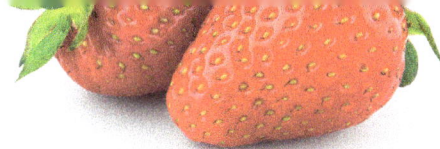

5-INGREDIENT FAMILY COOKBOOK

100 Easy, No-Fuss Recipes to Enjoy

— Kristen Smith, MS, RDN —

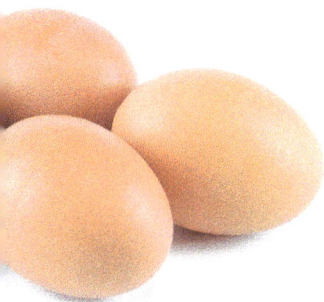

callisto
publishing
an imprint of Sourcebooks

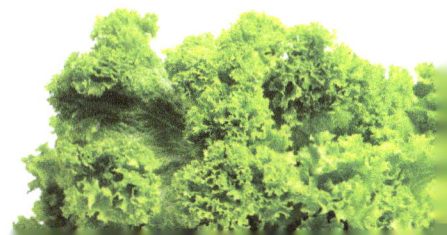

Copyright © 2021 by Callisto Publishing LLC
Cover and internal design © 2021 by Callisto Publishing LLC
Photography © 2021 Annie Martin, front cover (kebabs); © Annie Martin, p. vi; © Thomas J. Story, pp. x; © Hélène Dujardin, pp. 12, 118; © Darren Muir, pp. 24; © Elysa Weitala, pp. 45, 129, © Jennifer Chong, pp. 46; © Nadine Greeff, pp. 64; © Becky Stayner, pp. 94; all ingredients used under license from Shutterstock.com.
Author photo courtesy of Stephanie Madison.
Interior and Cover Designer: John Calmeyer
Art Producer: Hannah Dickerson
Editor: Anne Goldberg
Production Editor: Andrew Yackira
Production Manager: Michael Kay

Published by Callisto Publishing LLC C/O Sourcebooks LLC
P.O. Box 4410, Naperville, Illinois 60567-4410
(630) 961-3900
callistopublishing.com

Printed in the United States of America.

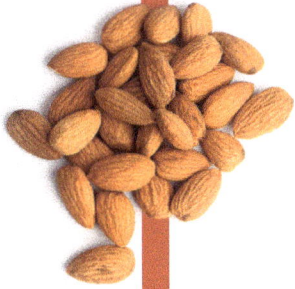

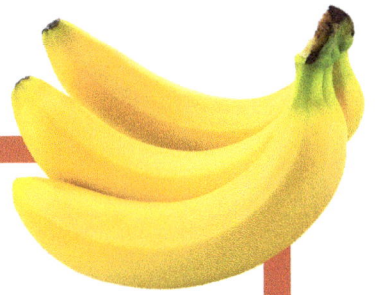

To my
FAMILY AND FRIENDS
who have always
SUPPORTED ME
and been
WILLING to TRY
my
culinary creations!

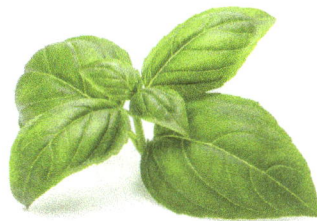

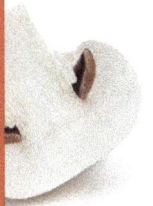

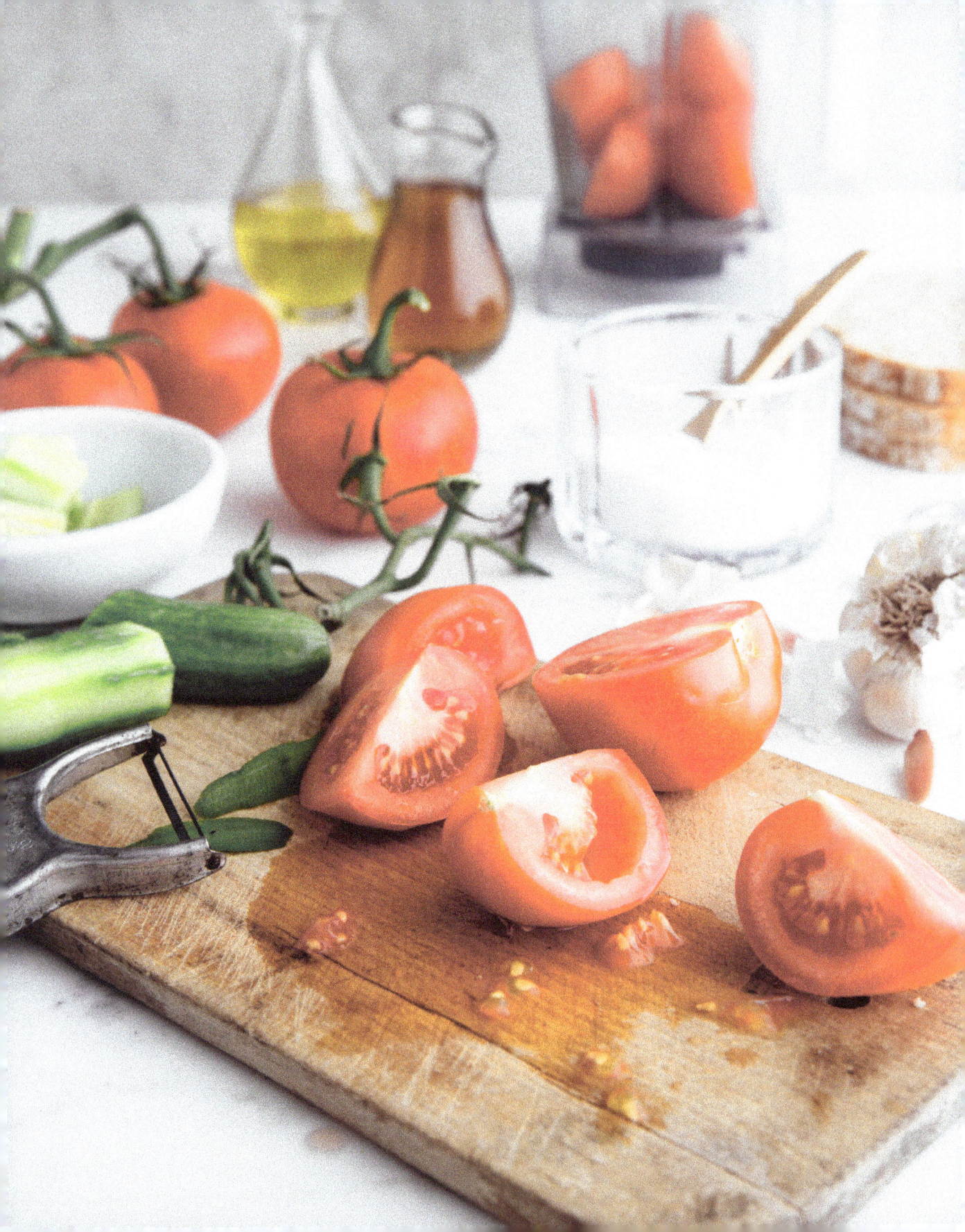

Contents

Introduction • viii

Chapter One
5-INGREDIENT FAMILY MEALS • 1

Chapter Two
BREAKFASTS • 13

Chapter Three
SOUPS AND SALADS • 25

Chapter Four
PASTA AND GRAIN MEALS • 47

Chapter Five
MEAT AND SEAFOOD MEALS • 65

Chapter Six
VEGETARIAN MAINS AND SIDE DISHES • 95

Chapter Seven
DESSERTS • 119

Measurement Conversions • 130

Index • 131

Introduction

Does this sound like your family?

It's 5:00 p.m., and you are dropping your oldest child off at soccer practice and headed to pick up your other two kiddos from after-school activities, only to then take them to piano lessons. Once each of these activities has ended, and you have all three children back in the car, you realize it's almost 6:45 p.m., and you have absolutely no plan for dinner. The children are in the back seat of the car complaining about how hungry they are. You see a fast-food chain a block away and quickly turn the car toward the establishment. Dinner is served.

You are definitely not alone if you don't frequently eat family meals together at the dinner table. The number of meals families eat together has drastically declined over the past several decades. It's not just unpredictable and busy schedules that make it difficult; differing food preferences and a lack of awareness of how to prepare a quick meal all present barriers to making this time happen on a regular basis.

It's no surprise that eating family meals together can offer numerous benefits to children of all ages. Meals eaten together allow families to converse and discuss the happenings of the day. Family meals allow parents to serve as role models and further promote healthy eating habits. Children who eat regular meals at the dinner table with other family members are more likely to eat fruits and vegetables and maintain overall nutrition habits.

While many of the impediments to eating meals as a family won't immediately go away, learning how to cook simple meals prepared with only 5 main ingredients that are still packed with flavor is essential when you do find time to gather together. This *5-Ingredient Family Cookbook* offers you 100 simple recipes to help ensure you can quickly prepare meals your entire family can enjoy around the table. The cookbook provides a variety of recipes, from breakfast and salads to meats and seafoods,

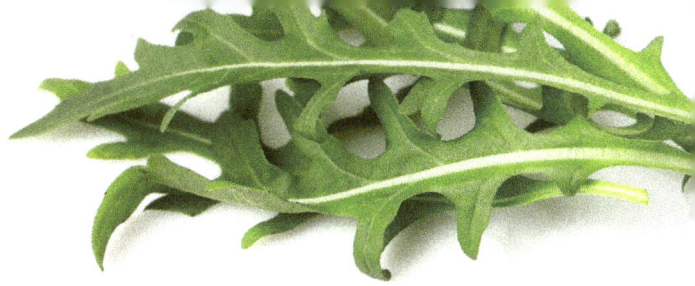

that are sure to be crowd-pleasers (try the Strawberry Cheesecake Toast on page 20 or the Sheet Pan Baked Fish and Chips on page 90). You are sure to find something for everyone in your family, including younger children who might be a bit more selective about their food choices. Hawaiian Pork and Pineapple Kebabs (page 83) is always a favorite for all ages!

If you feel overwhelmed when you start to think about preparing meals for your family, this book is for you. The recipes here can typically be prepared in 30 minutes or less from common ingredients you likely already have on hand. Get excited about spending less time at the grocery store! Wouldn't it be nice to save money by eating out less and cooking at home more? Whether you are feeding growing teenagers or active toddlers, your family will be blown away by these delicious recipes made with only five main ingredients. Who knows? Maybe takeout will become a thing of the past.

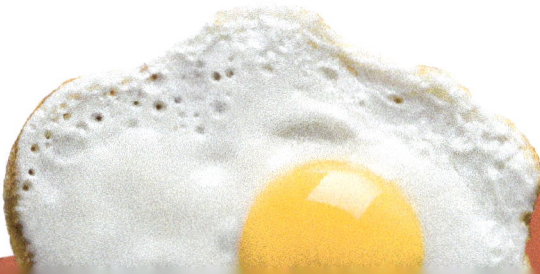

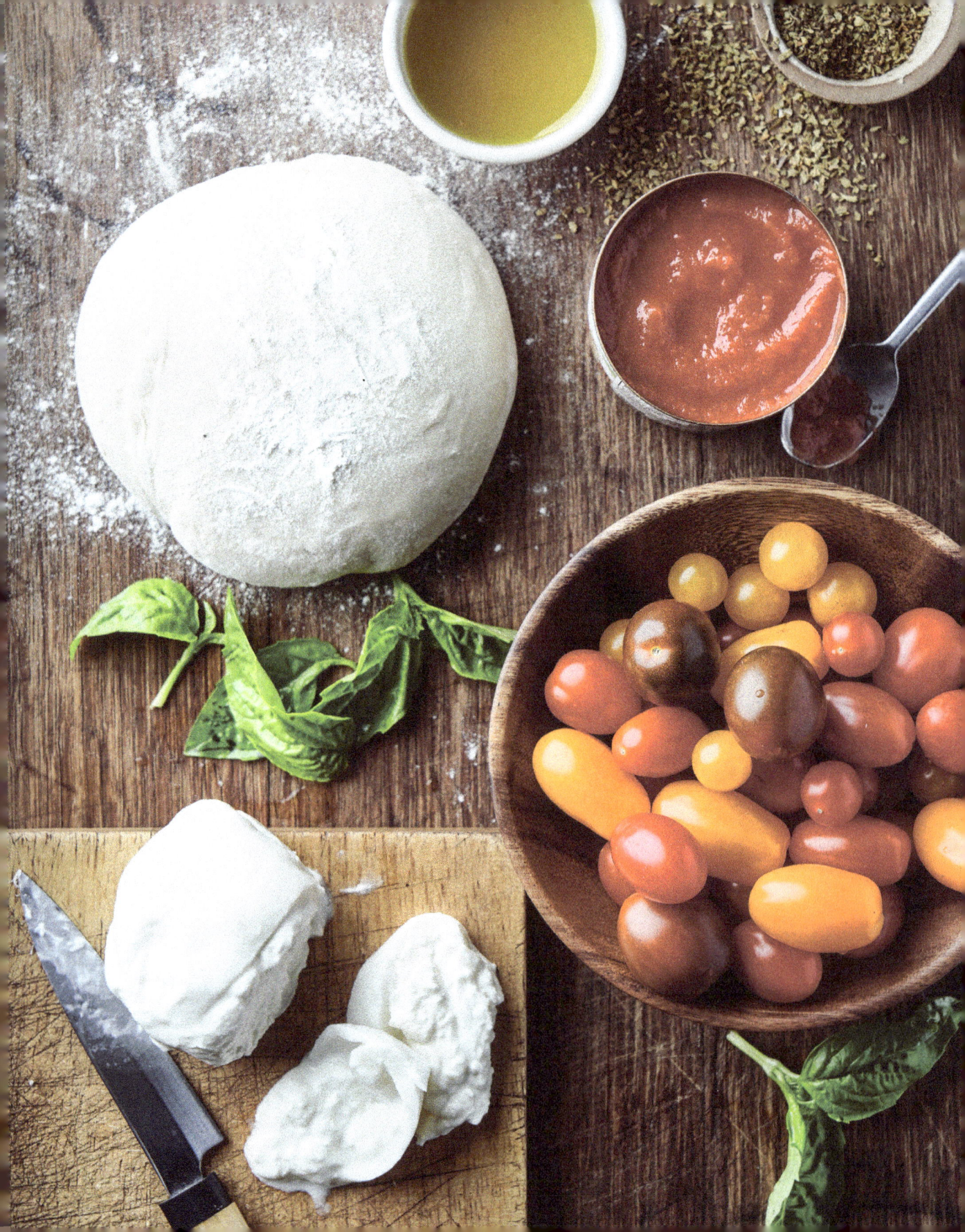

Chapter One
5-INGREDIENT FAMILY MEALS

Cooking can feel super intimidating if you have don't have a lot of experience. But the recipes in this cookbook are so simple, even the most amateur of chefs should be able to prepare them. Before you start preparing any of these recipes, make sure you are set up to succeed by reading the handy prep tips in this chapter and ensure you are stocked with the basic pantry staples listed on page 5.

Most people wouldn't believe 5-ingredient recipes could be as delicious as the recipes included in this book. But it's true! You are sure to gain confidence in the kitchen and motivation to prepare more family meals as you cook through this book and discover how flavorful they are. You will also feel good about feeding your family, because you'll be using healthy, wholesome ingredients. A win for all!

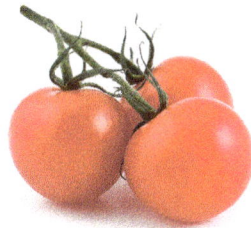

Easy Recipes Everyone Can Enjoy

A family meal together is even more impactful when the entire family eats the same meal. The goal is not to cook one meal for yourself, another for your partner, and then another for the children. By using this cookbook, which contains familiar ingredients, you will be able to simplify life and cook just one meal that everyone likes.

Busy families are more likely to want recipes that offer minimal preparation and even less cleanup. But they must taste great. Food does not need to be complicated to be full of flavor. It takes just a few basic ingredients like olive oil, a spice blend, fresh herbs, and citrus to elevate a recipe from blah to uh-mazing. Not only can simple cooking techniques such as roasting or sautéing enhance certain ingredients but they are also great methods for getting a meal on the table quickly.

One of the goals of this cookbook is to provide straightforward recipes that require only a few simple ingredients that are staples in your house or easily found at your neighborhood supermarket. No specialty food stores or online ordering should be required for these recipes.

Feeding a Family

With each new generation, how we feed our family seems to really shift. Today, it's likely you prepare fewer meals at home than your parents and grandparents did. You probably also serve more convenience and processed foods.

Time is one of the biggest challenges when it comes to feeding a family and ensuring that meals happen on a regular basis. Schedules are busier. More parents are working, and children are involved in more extracurricular activities. Multiple activities can mean different schedules and therefore different mealtimes. The result for most families is less time available to prepare meals and the inability to frequently enjoy meals together. For many families it just feels like survival!

Eating food not prepared at home can be an appealing option for many busy families. For those who live in large metro areas, it's incredibly easy to have food delivered or pick up takeout. It's really just a matter of clicking on an app, plus there is usually minimal cleanup. Enjoying a meal at a neighborhood eatery or restaurant might also be tempting; other than providing transportation to the establishment, there is minimal work involved on your part.

When it's so easy to get takeout or go to a restaurant, cooking wholesome, healthy meals can seem undesirable and intimidating. Often, this intimidation arises from a fast-paced lifestyle with little time to spend in the kitchen. Previous habits of eating less-nutritious foods, especially during childhood, may also play a role.

Also, for some families, finding healthy meals the whole family is willing to eat can be a challenge. Parents quickly find themselves preparing multiple dishes per meal and acting as a short-order cook in an effort to please everyone. Don't let this happen to you! The meals here are designed to appeal to the tastes of people of all ages.

The 5-Ingredient Solution

Keeping the ingredient list short is guaranteed to make cooking much more achievable and enjoyable. Five main ingredients really can create a variety of meal combinations without sacrificing flavor. Other benefits include:

Easy shopping: Who doesn't love when they can get out of the grocery store in a timely manner? There is nothing worse than spending hours in the grocery store and leaving with so many items that they are falling out of your cart. The absolute worst is unloading them when you get home! That won't happen with these recipes.

Saving money: Eating and ordering out can be expensive. Cooking with simple ingredients helps you stick to a reasonable budget so that when you do choose to eat out, you are able to splurge a little.

Saving time: Some of these recipes take so little time to make that it is actually quicker to cook than to order takeout and pick it up or have it delivered.

Better health: When you prepare your own meals, you have full control over the ingredients used. When you eat takeout or go to a restaurant, you have less control over the preparation of the food, including the amount of added fats and sodium and many other aspects that over time may contribute to poorer health status.

Sense of accomplishment: It's a great feeling to eat something that you made yourself. Don't be afraid to get the kiddos involved, too! It might even get a selective eater to try something new because they helped with the preparation and made it with their own hands. Learning to cook is a valuable and practical skill.

Fresh and Whole Foods

In addition to the four pantry staples mentioned on page 5, this book emphasizes dozens of whole, fresh foods. Many of these ingredients are commonly found in household refrigerators and pantries and will be familiar to most people. While there is no official definition of "whole foods," in this book it refers to foods in their whole, original state that have not been processed, such as fresh fruits and vegetables.

Whole foods are often less expensive than more processed ingredients, and they offer numerous nutritional benefits. Common examples include raw fruit, vegetables, and whole grains. A food in its whole form can ensure you are getting all the vitamins, minerals, and other nutrients the food has to offer. In the case of processed foods, components of the food are often modified during processing, making it possible for nutrients to be lost. An example would be apple juice versus a whole apple. When an apple is juiced, the fiber is stripped away, and thus a health benefit is removed.

Many ingredients used in these recipes can be easily replaced with other ingredients you have on hand. Substituting cauliflower or string beans instead of broccoli is one example. You can easily substitute whole grains like farro or quinoa instead of using brown rice. Don't stress if you don't have exactly what is listed on hand—you probably already have a simple replacement in your fridge or pantry!

Limiting the recipes to 5 main ingredients does keep them extremely simple; however, don't be afraid to take a few additional shortcuts if it helps make things even easier. Purchasing precut vegetables like broccoli florets or zucchini noodles for recipes such as Easy Tofu and Broccoli Stir-Fry (page 96) and Summer Squash "Pasta" with Peas (page 113) can save significant time. You might even consider canned or frozen vegetables when you are in a pinch. Preshredded cheese or pre-minced garlic might also save some time. Anything that can cut down meal preparation will help busy home cooks.

It's important to note that although this book emphasizes whole foods because they often offer less-expensive options with greater health advantages, you will also find a few quality, minimally processed convenience foods listed. Ingredients such as canned vegetables, salsa, and store-prepared pizza crust are occasionally suggested to simplify recipes without sacrificing flavor and help make recipe preparation that much easier for busy families. Plus, many of the convenience foods used in this book

PANTRY STAPLES EVERY COOK NEEDS

While the recipes in this book all contain only five main ingredients, there are a few pantry staples that you'll see regularly popping up. The four everyday items referred to as "pantry staples" in this cookbook are found in most of the recipes and are impossible to cook without. For easy reference, these staples are listed separately in each recipe.

The good news is that you most likely already have the pantry staples in your kitchen. Even if you don't, they are inexpensive options and typically have a long shelf life. For greater savings, buy them in bulk and you won't need to add them to your shopping list again any time soon.

Cider vinegar: This ingredient offers bold flavor with just a few calories when compared to other dressings and marinades. Typically sold as apple cider vinegar, it has a fruity, tart flavor.

Olive oil: This fat offers many health benefits and is great to use when sautéing or panfrying food. Also, it is an important ingredient for making great salad dressings. Extra-virgin olive oil has a fruitier flavor and is a bit more expensive; it's not essential to buy extra-virgin, but it can be excellent in dressings. If you want to minimize your expenses, normal olive oil is fine for everyday cooking.

Salt and black pepper: Seasonings are indispensable for enhancing food, and these two are the undisputed heroes. Salt and black pepper are classic, quality ingredients that can significantly enhance the flavor of food without overpowering it. A great technique is to season lightly when cooking and let each diner add more salt and black pepper to suit their own taste.

are likely items you already have in your kitchen, such as canned diced tomatoes and frozen spinach. But if time allows, the whole-food version will work in all the recipes in this book. For example, fresh vegetables can be used in any of the recipes that call for frozen or canned. And of course, feel free to use homemade salsa or tomato sauce, which work excellently in any recipes that call for the store-bought versions.

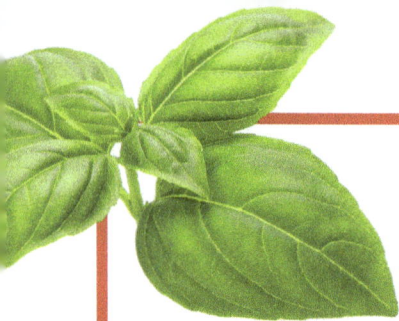

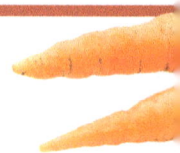

PLANNING OUT YOUR (FAMILY'S) WEEK

Mealtimes can be overwhelming if you don't have a plan. For many busy families, when the clock strikes six, they find themselves asking, "What's for dinner tonight?" This last-minute decision-making can lead to serving your family takeout or a freezer meal. However, if your priority is to serve your family a balanced meal that includes a lean protein, whole grains, fruits, and vegetables, meal planning with be a lifesaver for you. An added bonus of meal planning—it can save you money!

Think you don't have time for meal planning? Think again. Spending just a few minutes one day each week to plan your family's meals in advance can actually save you time throughout the week. Let's also be clear that meal planning can include eating some meals outside the house, but hopefully the focus will be on preparing home-cooked meals for your family.

Meal planning might seem overwhelming and time consuming at first. Here are some tips to get started and make things easier:

Start small. Start by planning for a few meals a week and work up to more as you get the hang of it. Planning for a week in advance works for most families, but over time you will find what works best for you and your family.

Put it in writing and make a shopping list. It won't feel official if you don't document it. Find an app on your phone or grab an old-school pencil and a sheet of paper and map out what your meal plan is for the week. Once you have established the plan, create a shopping list of any food items you don't have on hand that you will need to complete your plan.

Include everyone in the planning. Don't put all the pressure of meal planning on yourself! Assign each family member a few meals to plan for each week. This will add excitement and anticipation for the upcoming meals, too!

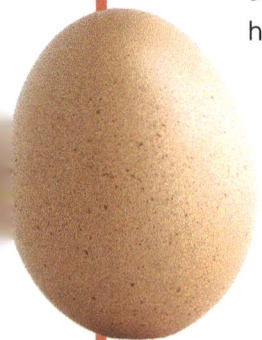

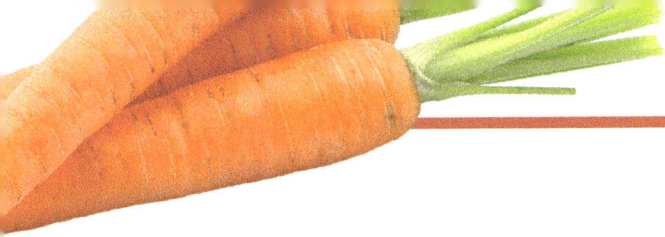

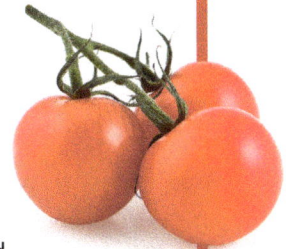

Meal prep. Meal planning and meal preparation are two different things. Once you have your plan finalized, make a list of any components of a recipe that might be prepared in advance that will save you time or make things easier when you actually start cooking. Do you need to thaw the chicken? Can you chop the vegetables earlier in the week when you have more time? If you know it's going to be super busy leading up to mealtime, the more you can do in advance, the better.

Cook in batches and embrace the leftovers. As you plan your meals for the week, think about the activities and commitments your family might have and how that will affect mealtime. If you anticipate a certain afternoon or evening will be a bit busier, cook enough for two meals the day prior. For family members who might not be huge fans of leftovers, think of creative ways to repurpose them. Cut up leftover cooked chicken or beef and serve them in tortillas. Add precooked vegetables or pasta to soups or salads.

Take a few meals off. In order to maintain your meal plan, it helps to take a break during the week or on the weekend and order takeout or go to a restaurant. Make sure to include these breaks as part of your plan for the week. Do what's right for your family.

Try themed meals. Themed nights can make meal planning a lot more fun for everyone. Create a vegetarian meal for "Meatless Mondays" or add "Taco Tuesdays" to your meal plan. The options for themed meals are nearly endless.

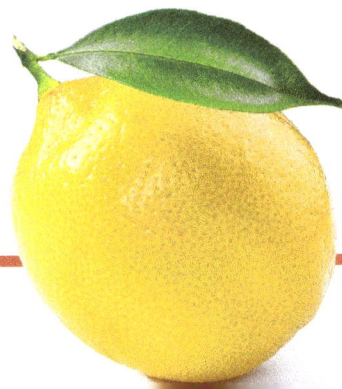

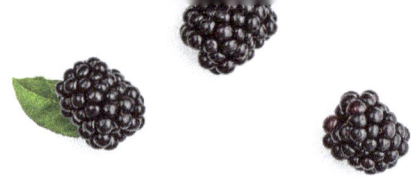

Sample Weekly Meal Plan

	Day 1	Day 2	Day 3	Day 4	Day 5	Day 6	Day 7
Breakfast	Hearty Salmon Avocado Toast (page 18)	Baked Oat Banana Muffins—double recipe (page 19) Fresh strawberries	Baked Oat Banana Muffins (leftovers) Fresh raspberries	Chocolate-Avocado Smoothie (page 22)	Strawberry Cheesecake Toast (page 20)	Savory Breakfast Egg Muffins (page 16)	Simple Buttermilk Pancakes (page 23) Fresh blueberries
Lunch	Lemon Chicken Orzo Soup (page 28)	Arugula Shrimp Salad with Lemon Olive Oil (page 41)	California Veggie Barley Bowls (page 59)	Easy Tuna and Avocado Panzanella Salad (page 42)	Chicken and White Bean Chili (leftovers)	Spinach Salad with Eggs and Bacon (page 43)	Couscous with Lemon Chicken and Olives (page 62)
Dinner	MEATLESS MONDAY: Easy Baked Ziti Casserole (page 54) Strawberry, Spinach, and Mozzarella Salad (page 36)	TACO TUESDAY: Buffalo Cauliflower Tacos (page 106)	Soy-Marinated Flank Steak (page 77) with Garlicky Peas and Mushrooms (page 116)	Chicken and White Bean Chili—double recipe (page 33)	Roasted BBQ Turkey Drumsticks (page 71) with Crispy Baked Carrot Fries (page 111)	Order takeout	Super Easy Chicken Fried Rice (page 57) with Honey-Lime Fruit Salad (page 120)

	Day 1	Day 2	Day 3	Day 4	Day 5	Day 6	Day 7
Breakfast	Baked Egg and Sausage Breakfast Taquitos (page 15) Fresh strawberries	Yogurt Banana Split (page 21)	Hearty Salmon Avocado Toast (page 18)	Simple Buttermilk Pancakes—double recipe (page 23) Banana slices	Simple Buttermilk Pancakes (leftovers)	Simple Baked Black Bean Huevos Rancheros (page 14)	Hearty Salmon Avocado Toast (page 18)
Lunch	Sweet and Savory Butternut Squash Soup (page 26)	Roasted Veggie Salad with Feta (page 39)	Tortellini Soup with Italian Sausage and Baby Kale (page 29)	Simple Beef and Black Bean Chili— leftovers	Chopped Mediterranean Salad (page 38)	Pinto Bean and Spinach Quesadillas (page 105)	Easy Grandma Pie Pizza —leftovers
Dinner	MEATLESS MONDAY: Lentil Sloppy Joes (page 98) Chili Butter Corn on the Cob (page 117)	TACO TUESDAY: Shrimp and Avocado Tostadas (page 92)	Simple Beef and Black Bean Chili—double recipe (page 34)	Lemon-Dill Salmon Packet (page 89) Wilted Balsamic Spinach (page 115)	Order takeout	Easy Grandma Pie Pizza (page 102) with Baby Greens Salad with Beets and Goat Cheese (page 40)	Sunday Roast Chicken Dinner (page 70) Brown Sugar Apple Galette (page 127)

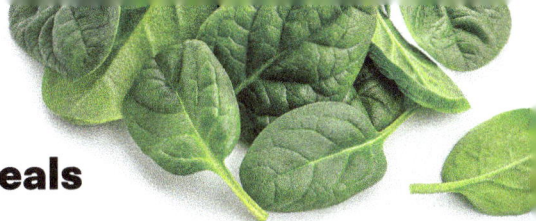

Use this Guide to Plan Your Meals

	Monday	Tuesday	Wednesday	Thursday	Friday	Saturday	Sunday
Activities for Day							
Breakfast							
Lunch							
Dinner							
Snacks							
Pantry Ingredients							
Food to Purchase							

Shopping List

Produce	Meat and Poultry	Canned/Pantry	Frozen	Dairy

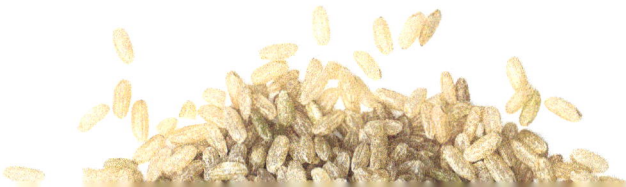

Essential Equipment

Another key to ensuring success in your kitchen is making sure you have the right equipment. Don't worry—fancy gadgets or electric appliances are not required to make these recipes. But a few simple necessities, which you might already own or can buy economically at stores like Target or Walmart, will ensure you're ready to hit the ground running. Here are the most helpful tools to have in your kitchen:

Baking/casserole dish: An 8- to 10-cup size works for the recipes in this book. The most commonly used shapes and sizes are 9-by-9-inch square or 11-by-7-inch rectangular, but you could choose rectangle, square, or oval and material such as glass, ceramic, or metal. A big benefit of baking dishes is that they serve as a vessel for baking or roasting your food while also acting as a serving dish.

Cast-iron skillet: Cast-iron pans are nearly indestructible and will evenly heat your ingredients and hold temperatures more consistently. Aim for a 12-inch skillet to best meet your needs.

Food thermometer: A thermometer made especially for food is essential for testing the doneness of meats and poultry. An instant-read option will make your life easier.

Knives and cutting board: A sharp 8- to 10-inch chef's knife and a paring knife are all you need. One large cutting board is sufficient, but you might consider at least two boards to keep meats and produce separate. A cutting board made from bamboo or other wood is the ideal material to help keep knives sharp and prevent your surface from getting too slippery.

Large pot with lid: A 6- to 8-quart pot is necessary for making family-size recipes of soups, stews, and some pasta.

Large skillet: A 10- to 12-inch skillet is perfect for recipes that serve 4 to 6 people. A basic stainless-steel skillet is ideal. It won't chip or stain like a nonstick skillet might. However, it's totally understandable if you feel the need to go the nonstick route for your skillet. For egg, pancake, or delicate recipes like fish, it will be easier to use a nonstick skillet.

Measuring cups and spoons: It's recommended to have both liquid and dry measuring cups on hand. For liquid varieties, glass options are both microwave-safe and sturdier. You can do plastic or stainless steel for the dry measuring cups, but you want to make sure they are durable and won't bend. Measuring spoons can be plastic or stainless steel.

Mixing bowls: A set of 3 mixing bowls with small, medium, and large sizes is helpful to meet the needs of all your recipe preparation. Aim for metal or glass options that look nice enough so they can also be used to serve food. Nesting options make for better storage.

Saucepan with lid: A small 2- or 3-quart pot is great for making sauces and grains.

Sheet pan: A large, rimmed 13-by-8-inch sheet pan is all you will need for basic roasting and baking. You will find yourself using a sheet pan for more recipes than you might expect.

Utensils: Lastly, don't forget a few essential utensils such as a heat-resistant silicone spatula, wooden spoon, whisk, handheld peeler, zester, and a colander for straining and draining. Keeping your kitchen stocked with these items will help you produce a higher-quality meal, and you will be more likely to have a more enjoyable experience in the kitchen (hopefully bringing you back for more!).

About the Recipes

The recipes in this book include useful labels to help you navigate the book. These include labels for **Quick Prep** meals that require only 15 minutes or less of hands-on preparation time before being cooked, recipes that can be both prepped and cooked in **30 Minutes or Less**, and meals that can be cooked in just **One Pot** or **One Pan**. There are also dietary labels for **Dairy-Free**, **Gluten-Free**, **Vegetarian**, and **Vegan** recipes.

Handy tips are also included to help you successfully cook the recipes. These include **Serving Suggestions** for accompaniments to serve with a meal, **Leftover Tips** for using any extra portions, **Cooking Tips** for how to improve your cooking, **Ingredient Tips** for how to select or use an item, and **Substitution Tips** for swapping out ingredients.

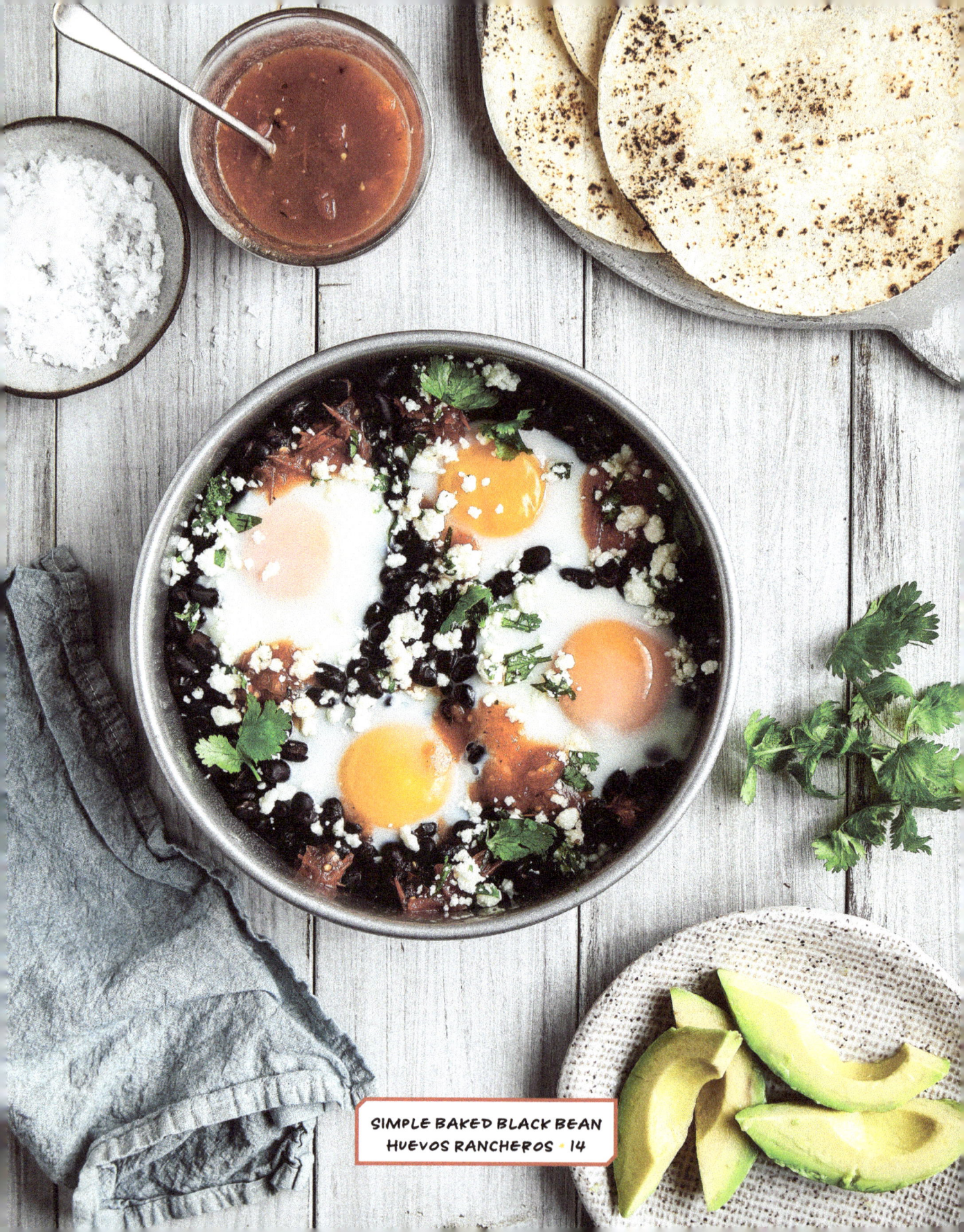

SIMPLE BAKED BLACK BEAN
HUEVOS RANCHEROS • 14

Chapter Two

BREAKFASTS

14 **Simple Baked Black Bean Huevos Rancheros**

15 **Baked Egg and Sausage Breakfast Taquitos**

16 **Savory Breakfast Egg Muffins**

17 **Sheet Pan Breakfast Bake**

18 **Hearty Salmon Avocado Toast**

19 **Baked Oat Banana Muffins**

20 **Strawberry Cheesecake Toast**

21 **Yogurt Banana Split**

22 **Chocolate-Avocado Smoothie**

23 **Simple Buttermilk Pancakes**

Simple Baked Black Bean Huevos Rancheros

PREP TIME *15 MINUTES*   COOK TIME *20 MINUTES*   SERVES *4*

GLUTEN-FREE   ONE POT   QUICK PREP   VEGETARIAN

This recipe is packed with flavor and will trick your family into thinking you spent hours preparing breakfast. The black beans are seasoned with salsa and paired with a silky sunny-side-up egg for a tasty and nutritious start to the morning.

Main Ingredients

2½ cups cooked black beans, drained and rinsed

¾ cup premade salsa, plus more for serving

4 large eggs

½ cup cotija cheese or queso fresco, plus more for serving

1 tablespoon chopped fresh cilantro

Pantry Staples

Nonstick cooking spray

2 tablespoons vegetable oil

Salt and black pepper

1. Preheat the oven to 400°F. Spray an 8- or 9-inch cake pan with nonstick cooking spray. Add the oil, beans, and salsa to the pan and stir until combined.

2. Gently create 4 wells in the beans. Crack 1 egg into each of the wells. Season each egg with a generous pinch of salt and pepper.

3. Place the pan in the oven and bake for 10 to 15 minutes, or until the egg whites are fully set but the yolks remain runny.

4. Let cool for at least 5 minutes. Sprinkle with additional cotija cheese, additional salsa, and cilantro. Divide the mixture between 4 plates and serve.

Ingredient Tip: If you can't find cotija or queso fresco cheese, you can use crumbled feta or shredded mozzarella instead.

Serving Suggestion: This recipe is delicious spooned into warmed tortillas and topped with sliced avocado.

Baked Egg and Sausage Breakfast Taquitos

GLUTEN-FREE   **QUICK PREP**

These baked taquitos offer all of the traditional breakfast fixings, like eggs, sausage, and cheese, tucked into a tightly rolled crispy corn tortilla.

Main Ingredients

6 uncooked sausage links

1½ cups chopped baby spinach

6 large eggs

2 cups shredded Mexican-style cheese, divided

12 (6-inch) corn tortillas

Pantry Staples

Nonstick cooking spray

Salt and black pepper

1. Preheat the oven to 425°F. Spray a large sheet pan with nonstick cooking spray and set aside.

2. Spray a large skillet with nonstick cooking spray and heat over medium heat. Add the sausage links and cook until all sides are browned, about 8 minutes total. Remove from the heat and cut the sausages crosswise into coins.

3. Add the chopped spinach to the skillet and sauté until wilted, 2 to 3 minutes. Return the sausage to the skillet with the spinach.

4. Crack the eggs into a small mixing bowl, add a pinch of salt and pepper, and whisk until combined. Add the eggs and 1 cup of cheese to the skillet and cook, stirring occasionally, until the eggs are cooked through and no longer runny. Remove from the heat.

5. Place the tortillas on a microwave-safe plate and microwave until they are extremely soft and pliable, 20 to 30 seconds.

6. Divide the egg and sausage filling equally between the tortillas. Top each with the remaining shredded cheese and roll up the tortillas tightly.

7. Place the filled and rolled tortillas on a sheet pan seam-side down. Bake for 10 to 15 minutes, or until they are crispy and lightly browned on top.

Savory Breakfast Egg Muffins

PREP TIME *10 MINUTES*   **COOK TIME** *22 MINUTES*   **SERVES** *4*

QUICK PREP

Breakfast egg muffins are an effortless savory recipe with traditional morning flavors. They take little preparation and can be customized with whatever foods you have on hand in the refrigerator and pantry. The best part about these egg muffins is they can be prepared in advance and quickly reheated for a complete and satisfying meal to start your day.

Main Ingredients

8 large eggs, whisked together

1 cup milk

1 cup shredded cheddar cheese

4 slices whole-wheat or white bread, torn into small pieces

3 to 4 slices deli ham, chopped

Pantry Staples

Nonstick cooking spray

Salt and black pepper

1. Preheat the oven to 350°F. Spray a 12-cup muffin tin with nonstick cooking spray and set aside.

2. In a small mixing bowl, mix together the eggs, milk, and cheese until combined. Season with salt and pepper.

3. Divide the bread pieces evenly between the muffin cups, filling them about ⅔ full. Sprinkle the ham pieces on top of the bread and pour the egg mixture over the top, nearly filling the muffin cups.

4. Bake for 18 to 22 minutes, or until the egg is no longer runny and set on top.

Substitution Tip: These egg muffins offer nearly endless options. To make them vegetarian, omit the ham and add a cooked vegetable of your choice. Or, replace the ham with other breakfast meats such as cooked bacon or sausage. For additional flavor, add cooked bell peppers.

Leftover Tip: To freeze leftovers, allow the muffins to cool completely. Arrange the muffins on a small sheet pan and place it in the freezer for 1 to 2 hours until frozen. Transfer the muffins to a resealable plastic bag and freeze for up to 3 months. To reheat, microwave on high for 30 to 60 seconds.

Sheet Pan Breakfast Bake

PREP TIME *10 MINUTES*   **COOK TIME** *30 MINUTES*   **SERVES** *4*

GLUTEN-FREE   ONE PAN   QUICK PREP

Making breakfast for your entire family has never been easier than with this mess-free and hands-off sheet pan recipe. Sheet pan meals are a magical answer for busy families with no time for preparation and cleanup in the kitchen. This flavorful sheet pan meal includes simple ingredients, and cooking everything together allows for each individual flavor to be absorbed into all the ingredients.

Main Ingredients

2 large potatoes, cut into ½-inch cubes

½ medium yellow onion, chopped

6 slices bacon, cut into fourths

4 large eggs

Pantry Staples

Nonstick cooking spray

1 to 2 teaspoons olive oil

Salt and black pepper

1. Preheat the oven to 400°F. Spray a large sheet pan with nonstick cooking spray. Arrange the potatoes and onion on the sheet pan and drizzle with olive oil. Add a pinch of salt and pepper. Mix them together well and spread them evenly over the sheet pan. Add the bacon slices in the gaps between the potatoes and onion.

2. Bake for 18 to 20 minutes, or until the potatoes are slightly browned.

3. Give the potato mixture a good stir with a spatula and create 4 wells. Carefully crack 1 egg into each of the wells. Sprinkle each egg with a pinch of salt and pepper. Bake for another 5 to 8 minutes, depending on whether your family prefers runny or firm eggs.

Cooking Tip: To keep the eggs from spreading too wide on the pan, create wells for each egg by pushing the potatoes and bacon toward the edges and middle. This will also allow the potatoes and bacon to continue cooking. Crack the eggs on a firm, flat surface such as your kitchen counter and carefully nestle them into one of the newly formed wells.

Hearty Salmon Avocado Toast

PREP TIME *10 MINUTES* **SERVES** *4*

30 MINUTES OR LESS **DAIRY-FREE** **ONE POT** **QUICK PREP**

Breakfast doesn't always have to be about bacon, eggs, or sausage. If your family is in need of a break from the traditional choices, offer them this recipe for avocado toast with salmon. The warm, crunchy toast is spread with a chunky avocado mixture and topped with a silky-smooth salmon piece—creating a flavorful morning meal option packed with nutritional benefits, which has never been easier!

Main Ingredients

2 avocados, pitted, peeled, and sliced

4 slices whole-wheat or white bread, lightly toasted

4 ounces smoked salmon, cut into slices

1 cup grape tomatoes, sliced

1 lemon, cut into wedges (optional)

Pantry Staples

Salt and black pepper

1. In a small mixing bowl, smash the avocados with a fork until they are well combined (some chunks are desired). Add a pinch of salt and pepper and mix well.

2. Spread the smashed avocado on one side of each slice of bread. Place 1 piece of smoked salmon on top of the avocado and top with grape tomatoes.

3. Sprinkle with a pinch of pepper. Squeeze a lemon wedge over each slice of toast, if desired.

Substitution Tip: No smoked salmon on hand? No worries! Substitute canned salmon or tuna.

Baked Oat Banana Muffins

PREP TIME *10 MINUTES*   **COOK TIME** *17 MINUTES*   **SERVES** *4*

30 MINUTES OR LESS   DAIRY-FREE   QUICK PREP   VEGETARIAN

These simple flourless muffins are naturally sweetened with bananas and contain only a small amount of added sugar. They have a cakelike consistency and are full of fiber, which will keep your family feeling full for the long haul.

Main Ingredients

1½ cups old-fashioned rolled oats

3 ripe bananas

3 large eggs

3 tablespoons maple syrup

1½ teaspoons baking powder

Pantry Staples

Pinch of salt

1. Preheat the oven to 350°F. Line a 12-cup muffin tin with muffin liners and set aside.

2. In a blender, combine the oats, bananas, eggs, maple syrup, baking powder, and salt and blend until the batter is smooth, 1 to 2 minutes.

3. Fill the lined muffin tins about ⅔ full with the batter. Bake for 13 to 17 minutes, or until a toothpick inserted into the center of a muffin comes out clean. Allow to cool for 5 to 10 minutes before enjoying.

Ingredient Tip: Look in your pantry for possible muffin toppings or additions. Sprinkle crushed or sliced nuts on top for an added crunch, mix in fresh fruit for added natural sweetness, or stir in dark chocolate chips for a sweet treat.

Leftover Tip: Store leftover muffins in an airtight container or resealable plastic bag in the refrigerator for up to 3 days.

Strawberry Cheesecake Toast

PREP TIME 10 MINUTES   COOK TIME 5 MINUTES   SERVES 4

30 MINUTES OR LESS   QUICK PREP   VEGETARIAN

This twist on a traditional French toast recipe offers a crunchy, buttery, sweetened toast topped with a dollop of vanilla Greek yogurt and fresh juicy strawberries. Greek yogurt serves as an excellent substitute for cream cheese in this recipe due to its rich flavor and creamy consistency. Your family has likely never had a toast quite like this one!

Main Ingredients

6 tablespoons butter

4 thick slices bread

Granulated sugar

1 (5.3-ounce) container vanilla Greek yogurt

1 cup sliced strawberries

Pantry Staples

Nonstick cooking spray

1. Spray a large skillet with nonstick cooking spray and heat over medium heat.

2. Spread butter on each side of the bread slices until well coated. Sprinkle each side of the bread with your desired amount of granulated sugar and place them in the skillet. Toast the bread until lightly browned, 1 to 2 minutes per side.

3. Allow the bread to cool for a few minutes. Top each slice with 2 to 3 tablespoons of Greek yogurt. Place the sliced strawberries on top and sprinkle with additional granulated sugar, if desired.

Substitution Tip: Put your own spin on this recipe by using another delicious fruit such as blueberries, raspberries, sliced kiwi, or cherries. Fresh, frozen, or canned versions of these fruits will work for this recipe.

Yogurt Banana Split

PREP TIME *10 MINUTES*   **SERVES** *4*

30 MINUTES OR LESS   GLUTEN-FREE   ONE POT   QUICK PREP   VEGETARIAN

Turn a family favorite dessert into a healthy and satisfying breakfast dish you can prepare in minutes. To enjoy the banana split as a breakfast option, skip the ice cream and use Greek yogurt instead. Greek yogurt adds a creamy texture and protein boost that is welcome on a busy morning. Preparing this breakfast recipe is incredibly easy—even the youngest of chefs can join in on the exciting preparation.

Main Ingredients

4 large bananas

2 cups vanilla or plain Greek yogurt

8 tablespoons fruit jam or preserves

Chopped nuts or mini chocolate chips, for topping

1. Peel the bananas and cut each one into 2 lengthwise slices. Arrange 2 banana slices on each of 4 plates. Spoon ½ cup of yogurt over each plate.

2. Drizzle 1 to 2 tablespoons of fruit jam or preserves over the yogurt and sprinkle with nuts, chocolate chips, or both.

Ingredient Tip: The topping choices for these banana splits are nearly endless. No need to purchase anything; simply survey your pantry for what you might have on hand, such as granola, oat cereal, nuts, or fresh fruit. For added sweetness, drizzle with a small amount of honey or maple syrup.

Chocolate-Avocado Smoothie

PREP TIME *10 MINUTES*   **SERVES** *4*

30 MINUTES OR LESS   GLUTEN-FREE   ONE POT   QUICK PREP   VEGETARIAN

If your family is in a breakfast rut, smoothies are an excellent option to change things up and still ensure your family is fueled for the morning. Smoothies are packed with flavor and can help boost nutritional intake. This one delivers a rich and creamy chocolate flavor your family will love! The avocados add an incredibly smooth texture without imparting any real flavor. (Don't worry, you won't feel like you are drinking guacamole!)

Main Ingredients

3 medium avocados, pitted and peeled

1 ripe banana

2½ cups milk

5 tablespoons unsweetened cocoa powder

¼ cup maple syrup

1. Combine the avocados, banana, milk, cocoa powder, and maple syrup in a blender and blend on low to medium speed until smooth, 1 to 2 minutes. You may need to stop the blender and scrape down the sides with a rubber spatula to ensure all ingredients are well blended.

2. Pour the mixture equally into 4 glasses and serve.

Serving Suggestion: Change up the presentation of the smoothie by serving it in a bowl instead of a glass. Smoothie bowls act as a canvas for a variety of toppings. Encourage your family members to choose nuts or seeds, fresh fruit, or chocolate chips and have them sprinkle them over the smoothie before eating with a spoon.

Simple Buttermilk Pancakes

PREP TIME *10 MINUTES* **COOK TIME** *20 MINUTES* **SERVES** *4*

30 MINUTES OR LESS **QUICK PREP** **VEGETARIAN**

Nothing says family breakfast like pancakes. Creating them from scratch might seem time-consuming in the morning, but this simple recipe will show you how easy it is to whip up a batch of pancakes whenever you want them. You will wonder why you have been relying on boxed pancake mix for so long!

Main Ingredients

2 cups all-purpose flour

3 teaspoons baking powder

2 tablespoons sugar

2 large eggs

2 cups buttermilk

1 to 2 tablespoons milk or water (optional)

Pantry Staples

¼ cup vegetable oil

Nonstick cooking spray

1. In a large mixing bowl, stir together the flour, baking powder, and sugar.

2. In a medium mixing bowl, whisk together the eggs, buttermilk, and oil. Add the wet ingredients to the dry ingredients and stir until just combined. The batter should be lumpy and slightly thick. If the batter appears to be too thick, you can add 1 to 2 tablespoons of milk or water and stir until combined.

3. Spray a large skillet with nonstick cooking spray and heat over medium heat. Spoon about ¼ cup of batter onto the heated skillet. Repeat until a few pancakes fit comfortably in the skillet (usually about 3, depending on the size of the skillet). Cook until small bubbles form around the edges of the pancakes, 2 to 3 minutes. Using a spatula, flip the pancakes and cook until browned, an additional 1 to 2 minutes.

4. Transfer the pancakes to a plate and repeat with the remaining batter.

Serving Suggestion: To create a complete balanced meal, serve the pancakes with a protein-rich food such as a side of eggs, bacon, or sausage and fresh fruit. Consider topping the pancakes with fresh fruit or adding it to the batter, or serve them warm with syrup or fruit preserves on top.

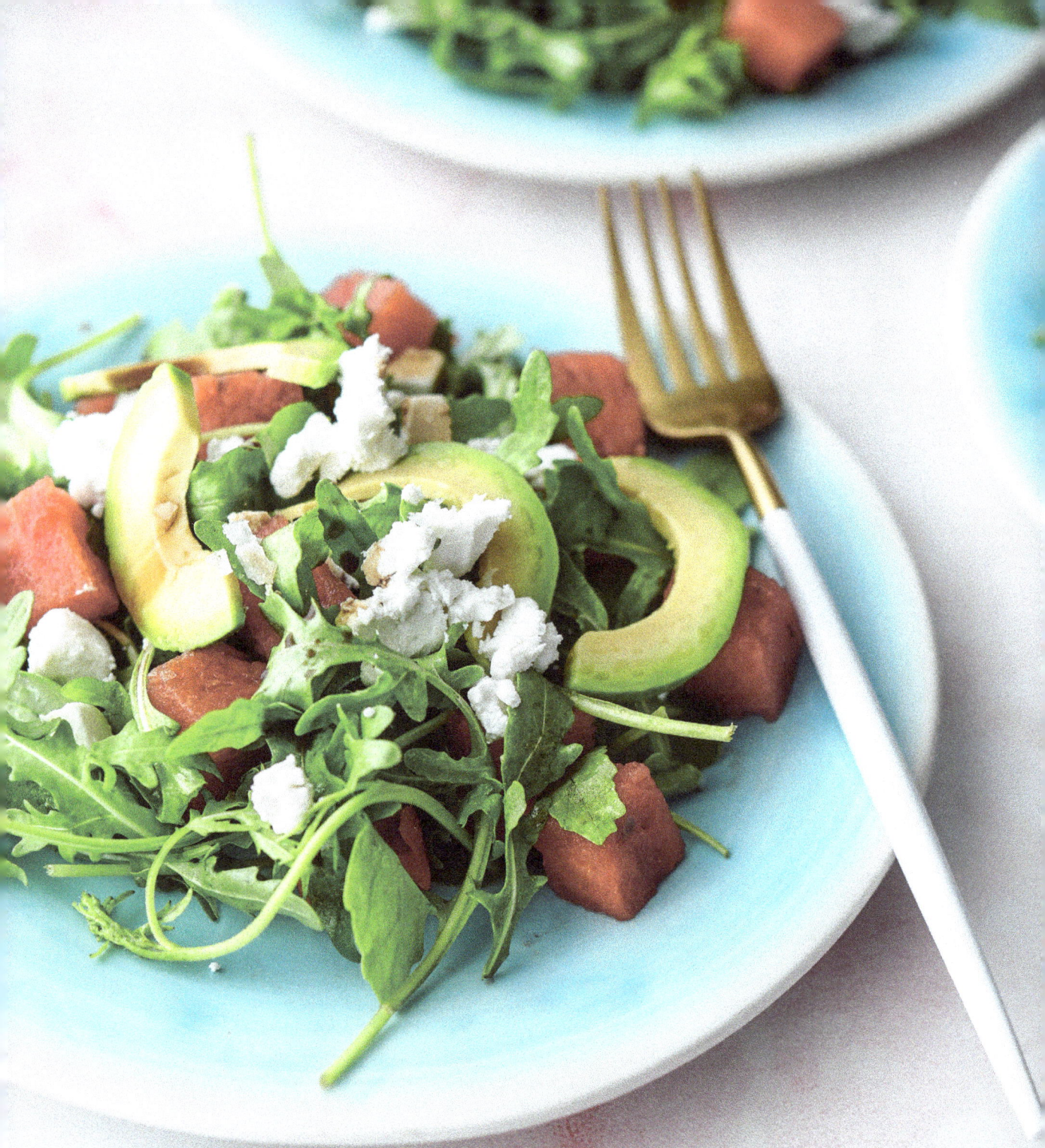

SUMMER ARUGULA SALAD
WITH WATERMELON · 35

Chapter Three

SOUPS AND SALADS

26 **Sweet and Savory Butternut Squash Soup**

27 **30-Minute Minestrone**

28 **Lemon Chicken Orzo Soup**

29 **Tortellini Soup with Italian Sausage and Baby Kale**

30 **Ham, Bean, and Potato Soup**

31 **Savory Chicken, Tomato, and Mushroom Stew**

32 **Smoked Sausage and Potato Stew**

33 **Chicken and White Bean Chili**

34 **Simple Beef and Black Bean Chili**

35 **Summer Arugula Salad with Watermelon**

36 **Strawberry, Spinach, and Mozzarella Salad**

37 **Caprese Corn and Tomato Salad**

38 **Chopped Mediterranean Salad**

39 **Roasted Veggie Salad with Feta**

40 **Baby Greens Salad with Beets and Goat Cheese**

41 **Arugula Shrimp Salad with Lemon Olive Oil**

42 **Easy Tuna and Avocado Panzanella Salad**

43 **Spinach Salad with Eggs and Bacon**

44 **Blue Cheese and Bacon Wedge Salad**

Sweet and Savory Butternut Squash Soup

PREP TIME *15 MINUTES*   **COOK TIME** *35 MINUTES*   **SERVES** *4*

GLUTEN-FREE   ONE POT   VEGETARIAN

This butternut squash soup is everything you would hope for. It is a bit sweet and a bit savory, and you can add some cayenne pepper to the bowl to make it a bit spicy, too. Although the ingredient list is simple, the result is a complex and rich flavor.

Main Ingredients

1 medium onion, diced

4 cups low-sodium vegetable broth or stock, plus extra, if needed

1 butternut squash, peeled, seeded, and cubed

2 tablespoons maple syrup

½ cup heavy cream

Pantry Staples

2 tablespoons olive oil

Salt and black pepper

1. In a medium soup pot over medium-high heat, heat the oil. Add the onion and sauté until translucent, 3 to 4 minutes.

2. Pour in the broth, add the squash, and stir until combined. Bring the mixture to a boil, reduce the heat to low, and simmer until the squash is tender and can be mashed, 20 to 25 minutes. Remove from the heat and let cool a bit. Using a masher, mash the pieces of squash and stir well.

3. Return the pot to the stove over medium heat. Stir in the maple syrup and season with salt and black pepper to taste. Stir constantly until the soup is smooth. Mix in the cream until blended. If the soup is too thick, more vegetable broth can be added to thin it out. Serve hot.

Cooking Tip: Butternut squash can be a bit difficult to cut. To make it easier, microwave the squash for 30 to 60 seconds. Make sure to use a sharp knife and a steady cutting board. Cut the ends off first, then peel the skin with a vegetable peeler. Cut the squash in half lengthwise and scoop out the seeds. You can now cut the big pieces into 1-inch cubes.

30-Minute Minestrone

PREP TIME *5 MINUTES*   **COOK TIME** *25 MINUTES*   **SERVES** *4*

30 MINUTES OR LESS   ONE POT   QUICK PREP   VEGAN

Minestrone is a hearty Italian soup made with beans and pasta. Some people make versions with ground beef or sausage, but this soup is vegan, so it is a perfect meal to make when one person at your table would like a meatless and dairy-free option. But if you'd like to add a meaty, robust flavor, feel free to toss in some chopped cooked bacon or pancetta when cooking.

Main Ingredients

6 cups vegetable broth

1 (14½-ounce) can petite diced tomatoes, Italian seasoned

1 (12-ounce) package frozen mixed vegetables

1 cup elbow macaroni

1 (15-ounce) can red kidney beans, drained and rinsed

Pantry Staples

Salt and black pepper

1. In a large pot over medium-high heat, bring the vegetable broth to a boil. Add the tomatoes and vegetables, stir until combined, and cook until the mixture comes to a simmer, about 5 minutes.

2. Lower the heat to low, add the macaroni and beans, and cook until the pasta is tender, 8 to 10 minutes. Stir well and cook until soup is heated through, another few minutes. Season with salt and black pepper and serve.

Ingredient Tip: Consider buying diced tomatoes that have an added element of flavor to them. In this recipe, canned tomatoes that have basil and garlic were used. If you can't find flavored tomatoes, you can always add a tablespoon of Italian seasoning along with the tomatoes when cooking the soup. Another way to add extra flavor is to replace vegetable broth with either beef or chicken broth. Keep in mind that if you make these changes, the soup will no longer be vegan or vegetarian.

Lemon Chicken Orzo Soup

PREP TIME *5 MINUTES*   **COOK TIME** *20 MINUTES*   **SERVES** *4*

30 MINUTES OR LESS   **DAIRY-FREE**   **ONE POT**   **QUICK PREP**

If anyone from your family is feeling under the weather, this soup might be the perfect solution. It's a simple chicken soup recipe made with short pasta and flavored with lemon juice for a tangy flavor. If lemon is not your thing, you can always leave it out. Feel free to add a vegetable like chopped carrots or spinach to make it a little heartier.

Main Ingredients

8 cups low-sodium chicken broth or stock

⅓ cup freshly squeezed lemon juice

1 cup orzo pasta

3 cups chopped cooked chicken

¼ cup chopped fresh parsley

Pantry Staples

Salt and black pepper

1. In a large pot over medium heat, combine the chicken broth and lemon juice and bring the mixture to a boil.

2. Add the orzo and chicken and cook until the orzo is tender, 8 to 10 minutes.

3. Stir in the parsley, season with salt and black pepper to taste, and serve hot.

Ingredient Tip: For a quicker preparation, use leftovers from a rotisserie chicken purchased at the grocery store or make the Sunday Roast Chicken Dinner (page 70).

Tortellini Soup with Italian Sausage and Baby Kale

PREP TIME 5 MINUTES   **COOK TIME 25 MINUTES**   **SERVES 6**

30 MINUTES OR LESS   ONE POT   QUICK PREP

Cheese tortellini make an excellent pantry or fridge staple. They cook up quickly, and you'll get food on the table fast. It's the perfect ingredient to use in a comforting pot of soup like this one. Italian sausage and baby kale are combined with the tortellini for a delicious soup.

Main Ingredients

12 ounces bulk Italian sausage or links with casings removed

8 cups low-sodium chicken broth or stock

1 (20-ounce) package fresh cheese tortellini, or a flavor of your choosing

5 to 6 ounces baby kale, chopped

Pantry Staples

1 tablespoon olive oil

Salt and black pepper

1. In a large soup pot over medium-high heat, heat the olive oil for 1 minute. Add the sausage and cook, breaking up the sausage with a wooden spoon, until it starts to brown and is no longer pink, about 10 minutes. Using a colander, drain the sausage of any extra grease and place the sausage back in the pot.

2. Add the chicken broth, lower the heat to medium, and bring to a boil.

3. Add the tortellini and cook until tender, about 5 minutes. Add the baby kale and cook just until it is wilted, 1 or 2 minutes more.

4. Season with salt and black pepper to taste and serve.

Substitution Tip: Baby spinach is a good substitution for kale in this recipe. It is as nutritious but has a milder flavor. Also, small refrigerated ravioli can be substituted for the tortellini. Just be sure to check the package cooking time as they will take a bit longer to cook.

Ham, Bean, and Potato Soup

PREP TIME *10 MINUTES*   COOK TIME *1 HOUR*   SERVES *6*

DAIRY-FREE   GLUTEN-FREE   ONE POT   QUICK PREP

There is nothing better than cooking a ham and being able to use the leftover bone in a soup like this one in the coming days. This simple soup made with ham, potatoes, and white beans and flavored with fire-roasted diced tomatoes will feel like a comfort food.

Main Ingredients

2 smoked ham hocks or 1 leftover ham bone, with some ham still attached

1 (14½-ounce) can fire-roasted diced tomatoes

1 (15-ounce) can white beans, drained and rinsed

1 (32-ounce) container low-sodium chicken broth

3 large potatoes, peeled and chopped

Pantry Staples

Salt and black pepper

1. Place the ham hocks or ham bone in a large soup pot. Add the chicken broth and about 3 cups of water to partially cover and bring to a boil over medium heat.

2. Lower the heat to low and simmer for 30 minutes.

3. Remove the ham hocks or ham bone and chop up any remaining meat. Place the meat back in the soup pot. Discard the bones.

4. Add the tomatoes, potatoes, and beans, stir until combined, cover, and cook, stirring occasionally, until the potatoes are tender, about 20 minutes. Add extra water, if necessary, to thin out the soup.

5. Season with salt and black pepper to taste and serve.

Substitution Tip: Several types of beans are great in this soup. Try kidney beans or black beans for a nice variation. If you don't have a leftover ham bone to use, you can always use smoked ham hocks or shanks. They can be found in the pork or smoked meat section of your grocery store.

Savory Chicken, Tomato, and Mushroom Stew

PREP TIME **10 MINUTES**   COOK TIME **35 MINUTES**   SERVES **4**

DAIRY-FREE   GLUTEN-FREE   ONE POT   QUICK PREP

This hearty chicken stew is perfect for your next Sunday supper or cozy winter meal. The combination of garlic, mushrooms, and tomatoes adds a bold, tangy flavor. It's great to prepare ahead; you can keep it warm until it's time to serve.

Main Ingredients

6 boneless, skinless chicken thighs, cut in half

3 garlic cloves, minced

1 pound white mushrooms, cut in half if large

1 (28-ounce) can crushed tomatoes

1 tablespoon dried Italian seasoning

Pantry Staples

2 tablespoons olive oil, divided

Salt and black pepper

1. In a large soup pot over medium-high heat, heat 1 tablespoon of olive oil. Add the chicken and sauté until it starts to brown, 3 to 4 minutes on each side. Transfer the chicken to a plate and season with salt and black pepper.

2. Lower the heat to medium and add the remaining 1 tablespoon of oil, garlic, and mushrooms and sauté until the garlic starts to turn golden, 2 to 3 minutes. Add the crushed tomatoes and place the chicken back in the pot. Add the Italian seasoning and 1 cup of water and stir until combined.

3. Bring to a boil. Lower the heat to low, cover, and let simmer until the chicken is very tender and the sauce is thickened, about 20 minutes.

4. Season with salt and black pepper to taste and serve.

Serving Suggestion: You can serve this stew over rice, pasta, or couscous. You can also serve with your favorite bread loaf or rolls. Bread serves as a delicious vehicle to dip into the sauce.

Smoked Sausage and Potato Stew

PREP TIME *15 MINUTES*   **COOK TIME** *30 MINUTES*   **SERVES** *4*

DAIRY-FREE   GLUTEN-FREE   ONE PAN   QUICK PREP

This sausage and potato soup is hearty and flavorful. Don't be afraid to try different types of smoked sausage for this recipe. Your grocery store will typically carry smoked beef or pork sausages, but smoked turkey and chicken sausage work as well. Any sausage you use will be delicious!

Main Ingredients

1 pound smoked sausage links, cut into 1-inch pieces

½ cup chopped onion

1½ pounds yellow potatoes, cut into bite-size pieces

2 cups low-sodium chicken broth or stock

6 ounces fresh baby spinach, roughly chopped

Pantry Staples

2 tablespoons olive oil   Salt and black pepper

1. In a large skillet over medium-high heat, heat the olive oil. Add the smoked sausage and onion and cook until the sausage starts to brown, 3 to 4 minutes.

2. Add the potatoes and chicken broth and stir until combined. Lower the heat to medium-low, cover, and simmer until the potatoes are tender, 15 to 20 minutes.

3. Add the spinach, stir until combined, and cook, uncovered, until the spinach is wilted and the sauce thickens.

4. Season with salt and black pepper to taste and serve.

Cooking Tip: You can make this dish up to a day in advance, or you could prep all the ingredients a few hours before cooking the dish. Keep them in a resealable plastic bag or container in the fridge until you are ready to cook.

Chicken and White Bean Chili

PREP TIME *10 MINUTES*   **COOK TIME** *25 MINUTES*   **SERVES** *4 TO 6*

DAIRY-FREE   **GLUTEN-FREE**   **ONE POT**   **QUICK PREP**

Canned white beans and cooked chicken meat are mixed with salsa verde in this lightened-up chili recipe. This not your standard beef chili recipe but keeps the ingredient list short and is a bit different and full of flavor.

Main Ingredients

1 pound chicken breast, cut into bite-size pieces

1 tablespoon chili powder

2 (15-ounce) cans white beans, drained and rinsed

1 (16-ounce) jar salsa verde

¼ cup chopped fresh cilantro

Pantry Staples

1 tablespoon olive oil

Salt and black pepper

1. In a large soup pot over medium-high heat, heat the olive oil. Add the chicken and cook, stirring occasionally, until browned, about 5 minutes. Add the chili powder and continue to cook, stirring occasionally, for about 4 minutes.

2. Add the beans and salsa verde and 3 cups of water. Stir until combined and bring to a boil. Lower the heat to low and simmer until the chili is slightly thickened and the chicken is cooked through, about 10 minutes.

3. Add the cilantro and season with salt and black pepper to taste. Serve with additional toppings, if desired.

Leftover Tip: Freezing chili is a great way to keep a good meal on hand for a busy night. This chili can be made as a double batch so you can also prep for a future meal. Store in an airtight container and freeze for up to 2 months. To reheat, just defrost overnight or defrost it in a microwave oven, then transfer the chili to a soup pot and reheat until bubbly and heated through, 10 to 15 minutes over medium heat.

Ingredient Tip: You can add any additional toppings like cheddar cheese, avocado, or sour cream to top it off, and serve in tortillas to make an easy fuss-free meal.

Simple Beef and Black Bean Chili

PREP TIME *5 MINUTES*   **COOK TIME** *35 MINUTES*   **SERVES** *4 TO 6*

DAIRY-FREE   **GLUTEN-FREE**   **ONE POT**   **QUICK PREP**

This chili recipe is made with only a few simple ingredients yet offers a traditional chili flavor. It's flavored with both jalapeño peppers and fire-roasted tomatoes to produce a delicious chili loaded with spice.

Main Ingredients

1 pound lean ground beef

2 jalapeño peppers, seeded and finely chopped

2 tablespoons chili powder

2 (14½-ounce) cans fire-roasted tomatoes with green chiles

2 (15-ounce) cans black beans, drained and rinsed

Pantry Staples

1 tablespoon olive oil

Salt and black pepper

1. In a large soup pot over medium-high heat, heat the olive oil. Add the ground beef and cook, stirring frequently, until browned, 5 to 7 minutes. Reserve 2 tablespoons of grease in the pot and drain the meat in a colander.

2. Add the jalapeños to the pot and sauté until soft, 4 to 5 minutes.

3. Add the cooked ground beef back to the pot along with the chili powder, tomatoes, and black beans and stir well until combined. Bring the mixture to a boil. Lower the heat to low, cover, and simmer until heated through, 15 to 20 minutes. If the chili mixture gets too thick, add a bit of water (¼ cup at a time) until it reaches your desired thickness.

4. Season with salt and black pepper to taste and serve.

Substitution Tip: Jalapeño peppers can be a bit spicy, so you can substitute a small finely chopped green bell pepper instead if you like.

Summer Arugula Salad with Watermelon

PREP TIME *15 MINUTES*   **SERVES** *4*

30 MINUTES OR LESS   **GLUTEN-FREE**   **ONE POT**   **QUICK PREP**   **VEGETARIAN**

This refreshing salad is perfect for warm temperatures. It combines sweet, salty, peppery, and fresh flavors into one delicious taste that is perfect for a light meal or a side dish.

Main Ingredients

6 ounces arugula

3 cups (¾-inch) cubed watermelon

½ cup crumbled feta cheese, plus more for topping

Juice of 2 limes

2 avocados, peeled, pitted, and sliced

Pantry Staples

½ cup olive oil

1 teaspoon salt

½ teaspoon black pepper

1. In a large mixing bowl, combine the arugula, watermelon, and feta.

2. In a small bowl, whisk together the lime juice, olive oil, salt, and pepper. Pour the dressing over the salad and toss until evenly coated.

3. Top the salad with the avocado slices and additional feta cheese, as desired. Serve immediately.

Ingredient Tip: You can add flavor to this recipe by tossing the watermelon and feta with chopped fresh herbs such as basil, mint, or dill. Use whatever suits your taste—you really can't go wrong.

Strawberry, Spinach, and Mozzarella Salad

PREP TIME *10 MINUTES*   **SERVES** *4*

30 MINUTES OR LESS   **GLUTEN-FREE**   **QUICK PREP**   **VEGETARIAN**

This sweet and salty salad makes for a refreshing meal on days when you feel like something light to eat. The strawberries and honey dressing provide a natural sweetness that, when combined with the salty, tangy flavor of mozzarella, is absolutely delicious. The crunchy sliced almonds are the perfect topping to the salad!

Main Ingredients

2 tablespoons honey

6 ounces fresh baby spinach

4 ounces fresh mozzarella balls, each cut in half

2 cups strawberries, cored and halved or quartered

⅓ cup toasted sliced almonds

Pantry Staples

3 tablespoons olive oil

2 tablespoons cider vinegar

½ teaspoon salt

Black pepper

1. In a small bowl, whisk together the honey, oil, vinegar, salt, and 1 tablespoon of water until well blended. Set the dressing aside.

2. In a large bowl, toss together the spinach, mozzarella, strawberries, and dressing. Transfer the salad mixture to a shallow bowl or a platter.

3. Sprinkle the salad with the almonds, add black pepper to taste, and serve.

Ingredient Tip: Select firm, unbruised, and fully ripe berries from your local grocery store or market. Strawberries will not continue to ripen once they are picked.

Caprese Corn and Tomato Salad

PREP TIME *10 MINUTES*   **COOK TIME** *10 MINUTES*
CHILL TIME *2 HOURS*   **SERVES** *4*

GLUTEN-FREE   **ONE PAN**   **QUICK PREP**   **VEGETARIAN**

Corn is combined with classic caprese salad ingredients including basil, tomatoes, and fresh mozzarella balls. The salad is incredibly simple to whip up and packed full of vibrant flavors. It's perfect for your next picnic or potluck dinner.

Main Ingredients

6 cups fresh or frozen corn

1 tablespoon minced garlic

⅓ cup chopped fresh basil

1 pound grape tomatoes or small cherry tomatoes, halved

8 ounces fresh mozzarella balls, halved

Pantry Staples

3 tablespoons olive oil, divided

1 tablespoon cider vinegar

Salt and black pepper

1. In a large skillet over medium heat, warm 1 tablespoon of olive oil. Add the corn and garlic and sauté until the corn is tender and the garlic begins to turn golden, 5 to 6 minutes.

2. Transfer the corn and garlic to a serving bowl and let cool slightly.

3. Add the basil, tomatoes, and mozzarella to the corn and mix well until combined.

4. In a small bowl, whisk together the remaining 2 tablespoons olive oil and the vinegar. Drizzle the mixture over the salad and gently stir until combined.

5. The salad can be eaten at room temperature, or cover and refrigerate for at least 2 hours. Season with salt and black pepper to taste and serve.

Cooking Tip: For easy kernel removal, hold an ear of shucked corn over a cutting board. With the end of the corncob on the board, cut down the side of the cob to remove the kernels. Rotate the cob and continue to cut until all the kernels are removed.

Chopped Mediterranean Salad

PREP TIME *10 MINUTES*   **SERVES** *4*

30 MINUTES OR LESS   GLUTEN-FREE   QUICK PREP   VEGETARIAN

Ordering a chopped salad in a restaurant can seem like a treat because someone else has to chop up the long list of ingredients. Luckily this salad contains only a handful of quickly prepped ingredients that come together in no time. Get the family involved in preparation and have them chop their own salads!

Main Ingredients

6 ounces chopped romaine lettuce

1 (15-ounce) can chickpeas, rinsed and drained

2 cups chopped tomatoes

¼ cup chopped kalamata olives

⅓ cup crumbled feta cheese

Pantry Staples

3 tablespoons olive oil

2 tablespoons cider vinegar

Salt and black pepper

1. In a small bowl, whisk together the olive oil and vinegar until well blended.

2. In a large bowl, toss together the lettuce, chickpeas, tomatoes, olives, and dressing.

3. Sprinkle with feta cheese. Season with salt and black pepper, if desired, and serve.

Serving Suggestion: For a heartier salad, top with a canned seafood option such as tuna in olive oil.

Roasted Veggie Salad with Feta

PREP TIME *15 MINUTES* **COOK TIME** *15 MINUTES* **SERVES** *4*

30 MINUTES OR LESS **ONE PAN** **QUICK PREP** **VEGETARIAN**

This is a perfect salad for a family meal or your next potluck dinner. Dressed with a simple apple cider dressing, it can be served warm, cold, or at room temperature.

Main Ingredients

1 large red pepper, seeded and chopped

2 large carrots, peeled and cut into bite-size pieces

1 medium zucchini, cut into 1-inch pieces

8 ounces orzo pasta

4 ounces crumbled feta cheese

Pantry Staples

4 tablespoons olive oil, divided

Salt and black pepper

2 tablespoons cider vinegar

1. Preheat the oven to 400°F. Line a large sheet pan with parchment paper or spray it with cooking spray.

2. In a large bowl, toss together the pepper, the carrots, the zucchini, 1 tablespoon of olive oil, and a dash of salt and black pepper.

3. Spread out the vegetables on the sheet pan and roast for about 15 minutes, or until the carrots are crisp but tender and cooked to your liking.

4. While the veggies are roasting, bring a large pot of salted water to a boil over high heat. Add the orzo and cook until al dente, 7 to 10 minutes. Drain and rinse under cold water.

5. In a large bowl, mix together the orzo and roasted veggies (including the pan juices). Add the feta cheese, the remaining 3 tablespoons of olive oil, and the cider vinegar and toss well.

6. Serve the salad warm, at room temperature, or chilled.

Substitution Tip: To make this salad dairy-free and vegan, omit the feta cheese and substitute one pitted, peeled, and diced avocado. Avocado has a nice creaminess, making it a great substitute for cheese.

Baby Greens Salad with Beets and Goat Cheese

PREP TIME *10 MINUTES*   **SERVES** *4*

30 MINUTES OR LESS   GLUTEN-FREE   QUICK PREP   VEGETARIAN

This salad tastes like something fancy you might order in a restaurant, but it's super simple to make. The earthy flavor of beets goes well with the creamy cheese, and a touch of honey makes the dressing especially delicious. If you want an extra crunch to the salad, you can sprinkle it with some chopped walnuts.

Main Ingredients

2 tablespoons honey

6 ounces baby greens or mesclun salad mix

2 cups sliced cooked beets, drained (canned or vacuum packed)

4 ounces crumbled goat cheese

Pantry Ingredients

3 tablespoons olive oil

2 tablespoons cider vinegar

Salt and black pepper

1. In a small bowl, whisk together the honey, olive oil, vinegar, and 1 tablespoon of water. Set aside.

2. In a large bowl, toss together the baby greens and the dressing. Arrange the salad on a large deep plate. Top with the beets and sprinkle with the goat cheese, season with salt and black pepper to taste, and serve.

Substitution Tip: Feta cheese makes a great substitution for goat cheese. It is saltier, so make sure to adjust the salt and black pepper to taste.

Arugula Shrimp Salad with Lemon Olive Oil

PREP TIME *10 MINUTES*   **COOK TIME** *5 MINUTES*   **SERVES** *4*

30 MINUTES OR LESS   **DAIRY-FREE**   **GLUTEN-FREE**   **ONE PAN**   **QUICK PREP**

You will be surprised by how so few ingredients can produce such a mouth-watering and satisfying salad! This arugula salad with shrimp and grape tomatoes is topped with a refreshing lemon oil dressing.

Main Ingredients

12 ounces large cooked shrimp, deveined and tails removed

Juice of 1 small lemon

5 to 6 ounces baby arugula

2 cups grape tomatoes, halved

Pantry Staples

4 tablespoons olive oil, divided

½ teaspoon salt, plus more if desired

Black pepper

1. In a medium skillet over medium-high heat, heat 1 tablespoon of olive oil. Add the shrimp and cook until they are cooked through and no longer pink, 5 to 6 minutes. Transfer the shrimp to a bowl and set aside to cool.

2. In a small bowl, whisk together the lemon juice, the remaining 3 tablespoons of olive oil, and the salt and set aside.

3. In a large bowl, toss together the arugula, the tomatoes, and half the dressing. Top with the shrimp.

4. Drizzle the remaining dressing on top of the shrimp and season with salt and black pepper to taste. Serve immediately.

Ingredient Tip: Keep bags of frozen peeled and deveined shrimp in your freezer. When ready to cook, defrost them by placing them in a colander and running cold water over them for about 10 minutes.

Easy Tuna and Avocado Panzanella Salad

PREP TIME *15 MINUTES*   **COOK TIME** *15 MINUTES*   **SERVES** *4*

30 MINUTES OR LESS   DAIRY-FREE   QUICK PREP

This hearty salad features bread cubes, white tuna, and cherry tomatoes. Panzanella, or "bread salad," is a delicious solution to stale bread you might have on hand. With a Panzanella salad, the bread soaks up all the delicious juices of many of the ingredients, like the tomatoes and dressing.

Main Ingredients

2 cups cherry tomatoes, halved

1 (5-ounce) can chunk white tuna in oil, drained and flaked

1 avocado, pitted, peeled, and diced

3 cups Italian bread cubes

4 cups chopped romaine lettuce

Pantry Ingredients

4 tablespoons olive oil

2 tablespoons cider vinegar

Salt and black pepper

1. Preheat the oven to 325°F. Line a large sheet pan with parchment paper or spray it with cooking spray.

2. In a large bowl, whisk together the olive oil, vinegar, and a dash of salt and black pepper. Add the tomatoes, tuna, and avocado and stir until combined. Let sit for 10 minutes.

3. Spread out the bread cubes on the sheet pan and bake for 10 to 15 minutes, or until the bread is lightly toasted.

4. Add the toasted bread cubes and romaine lettuce to the bowl and mix well. Season with salt and black pepper to taste and serve.

Spinach Salad with Eggs and Bacon

PREP TIME *10 MINUTES*   SERVES *4*

30 MINUTES OR LESS   GLUTEN-FREE   QUICK PREP

Bacon's salty and smoky flavor is a delicious addition to this spinach salad, which also includes eggs for a substantial and satisfying lunch or dinner.

Main Ingredients

10 to 12 ounces fresh baby spinach

1 small red onion, thinly sliced

2 cups grape tomatoes, halved

6 slices cooked bacon, crumbled

4 hard-boiled eggs, sliced

Pantry Ingredients

¼ cup olive oil

2 tablespoons cider vinegar

½ teaspoon salt

¼ teaspoon black pepper

1. In a small bowl, whisk together the olive oil, vinegar, salt, and black pepper until well blended.

2. In a large bowl, toss together the spinach, onion, tomatoes, and bacon. Add the dressing and toss until evenly coated. Transfer the salad to a large platter, top with the sliced eggs, and serve.

Cooking Tip: For convenience, you may choose to go with pre-boiled eggs, which are available in most grocery stores. If you prefer to cook your own, the process is fairly simple. Place the raw eggs in a medium pot and fill with water to 1 inch above the eggs. Bring to a boil over medium-high heat. Remove the pot from the heat and let the eggs sit in the pot for 10 to 12 minutes. Drain and transfer to an ice-water bath to cool. The eggs can be kept in the refrigerator for up to one week.

Blue Cheese and Bacon Wedge Salad

PREP TIME *10 MINUTES*   **SERVES** *4*

30 MINUTES OR LESS   **GLUTEN-FREE**   **QUICK PREP**

There is nothing better than a cold, crispy wedge of lettuce topped with bacon, blue cheese, juicy, ripe tomatoes, and balsamic glaze. Wedge salads are often served at steakhouses but are incredibly simple to make at home with a few simple ingredients, including iceberg lettuce!

Main Ingredients

½ large head iceberg lettuce

4 slices cooked bacon, crumbled

1 cup chopped tomatoes

¼ cup crumbled blue cheese

4 to 6 tablespoons balsamic glaze

1. Remove the outer leaves and stem from the lettuce. Cut the lettuce into 4 wedges.

2. Place each wedge on a plate and top with the crumbled bacon, tomatoes, and blue cheese.

3. Drizzle each salad with 1 tablespoon of balsamic glaze (adding more as desired) and serve.

Ingredient Tip: Balsamic glaze is sold in most grocery stores, but if you can't find it, you can always make your own. Just cook down 1 cup of balsamic vinegar on low heat until it is reduced by half. This will take 15 to 20 minutes. You will have a delicious sweet and tangy glaze that can be stored in a glass jar in your refrigerator for up to 2 months.

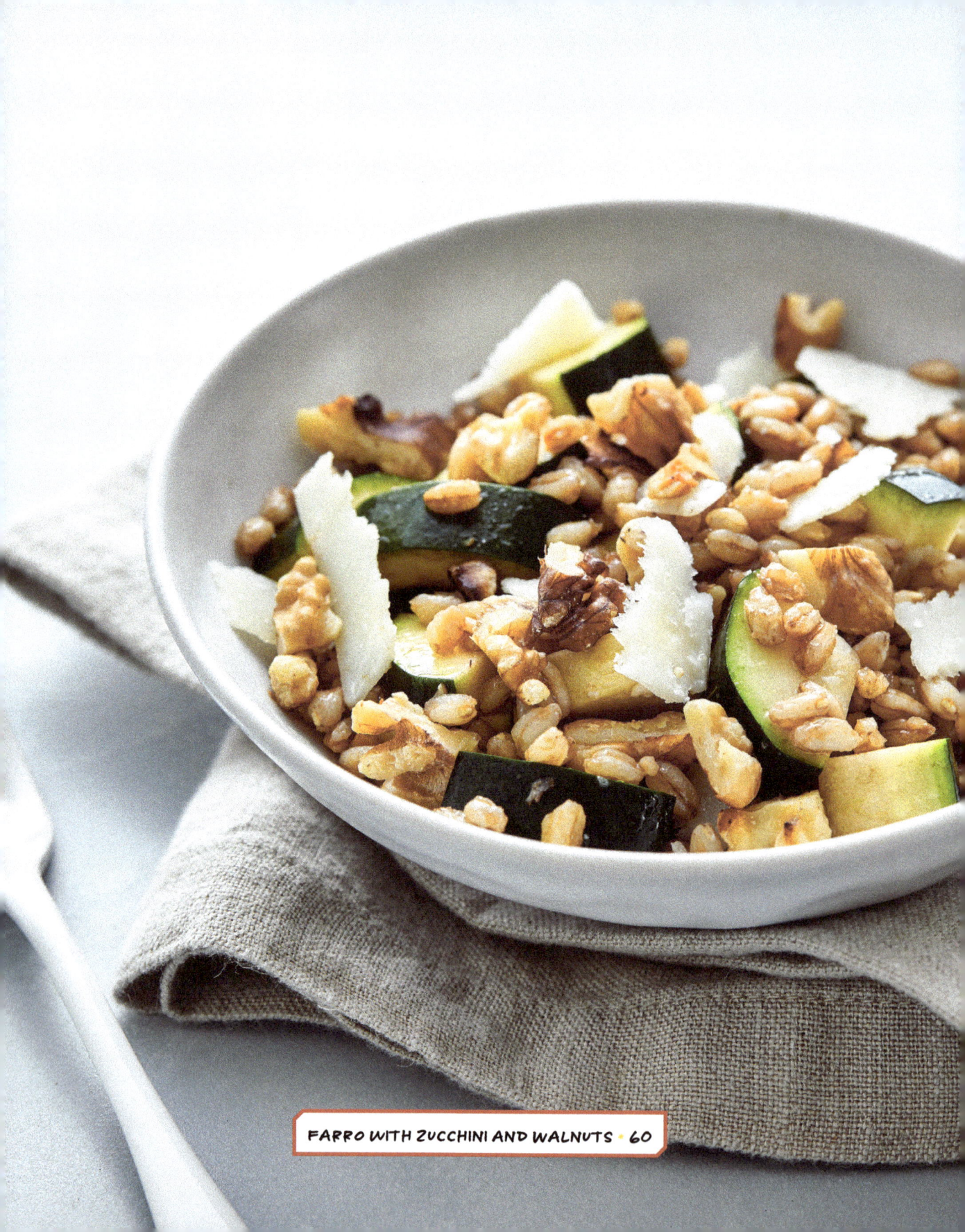
FARRO WITH ZUCCHINI AND WALNUTS • 60

Chapter Four

PASTA AND GRAIN MEALS

48 **Tomato-Basil Gnocchi**

49 **Spicy Peanut Noodles**

50 **Black Pepper Spaghetti with Garlic and Parmesan**

51 **Easiest Baked Mac and Cheese**

52 **Penne with Broccoli Pesto**

53 **Shrimp Orzo Skillet**

54 **Easy Baked Ziti Casserole**

55 **Penne Florentine with Bacon**

56 **Rigatoni with Sausage and Chunky Tomato Sauce**

57 **Super Easy Chicken Fried Rice**

58 **Easiest Butternut Squash Risotto**

59 **California Veggie Barley Bowls**

60 **Farro with Zucchini and Walnuts**

62 **Couscous with Lemon Chicken and Olives**

63 **Quinoa with Spicy Black Beans and Sausage**

Tomato-Basil Gnocchi

PREP TIME **5 MINUTES**   COOK TIME **20 MINUTES**   SERVES **4**

30 MINUTES OR LESS   ONE POT   QUICK PREP   VEGETARIAN

These two simple ingredients, tomatoes and basil, are a flavorsome combination—even the smell is intoxicating. Both can be easily grown at home with limited space but are also easily accessible at your local supermarket. Toss them with pillows of gnocchi, and the result will be a flavorful meal the whole family will love.

Main Ingredients

1 (16-ounce) package potato gnocchi

2 garlic cloves, minced

3 large plum tomatoes, chopped

3 tablespoons finely chopped fresh basil, plus extra for garnish

⅓ cup shredded vegetarian Parmesan cheese, plus extra for serving

Pantry Staples

2 tablespoons olive oil

Salt and black pepper

1. Bring a large pot of water to a boil over high heat. Add the gnocchi and cook until they are al dente and float to the top of the pot, 2 to 4 minutes. Reserve ½ cup of pasta water and drain the gnocchi in a colander.

2. In the same pot over medium heat, combine the olive oil and garlic and cook until the garlic starts to sizzle. Add the tomatoes and bring the mixture to a simmer. Cover and cook for 5 minutes.

3. Add the gnocchi, basil, and reserved pasta water to the pan and simmer, stirring occasionally, until the sauce is thickened, 5 to 10 minutes. Season with salt and black pepper to taste.

4. Transfer the mixture to a medium bowl and toss with the Parmesan cheese. Garnish with extra basil if desired and serve.

Ingredient Tip: Gnocchi can be purchased frozen in bags or in shelf-stable packages in the pasta section of your grocery store. Cook them just like pasta in boiling water. Make sure not to overcook, or they will become gummy.

Spicy Peanut Noodles

PREP TIME _10 MINUTES_   **COOK TIME** _20 MINUTES_   **SERVES** _6_

30 MINUTES OR LESS   **DAIRY-FREE**   **QUICK PREP**   **VEGAN**

Most people don't think of peanut butter for pasta sauces, but when paired with a few other simple ingredients, it can create a delectable sauce. Restaurants usually use rice noodles in a pasta dish with peanut sauce, but linguine can be easier to cook and serve as leftovers.

Main Ingredients

1 (16-ounce) package linguine

1 (16-ounce) package coleslaw mix

2 tablespoons soy sauce

½ cup peanut butter

2 to 3 tablespoons chili garlic sauce

Pantry Staples

1 tablespoon olive oil

Salt and black pepper

1. Bring a large pot of salted water to a boil over high heat. Add the linguine and cook until al dente, about 8 minutes. Reserve ⅓ cup of the pasta water and drain the linguine.

2. In a large skillet over medium-high heat, heat the olive oil. Add the coleslaw mix and ½ teaspoon salt and cook, stirring, until soft, 5 to 7 minutes.

3. In a small bowl, whisk together the soy sauce, the peanut butter, 2 to 3 tablespoons chili garlic sauce (depending on how spicy you like it), and the reserved pasta water.

4. Using tongs, add the linguine to the coleslaw mix. Add the peanut sauce and toss until combined. If necessary, add a little bit more water to thin out the sauce.

5. Season with salt and black pepper to taste and serve.

Leftover Tip: These noodles are delicious as a cold lunch the next day. To change up the flavor profile, add a spoonful or two of cider vinegar and some chopped red bell pepper.

Black Pepper Spaghetti with Garlic and Parmesan

PREP TIME 10 MINUTES   COOK TIME 20 MINUTES   SERVES 6

30 MINUTES OR LESS   ONE POT   QUICK PREP   VEGETARIAN

Pasta dishes can be prepared quickly and offer a blank canvas for endless meal opportunities. For example, with this simple, vegetarian garlic and Parmesan pasta meal, it's easy to add a vegetable or a protein such as chicken, meat, or fish to make it heartier and appealing to omnivores.

Main Ingredients

1 (16-ounce) package spaghetti

4 tablespoons butter

3 garlic cloves, minced

½ cup grated vegetarian Parmesan cheese, plus extra for serving

Pantry Ingredients

2 teaspoons black pepper

1. Bring a large pot of water to a boil over medium-high heat. Add the spaghetti and cook until al dente, or according to the package instructions, 6 to 8 minutes. Reserve ⅔ cup of the pasta water and drain the spaghetti. Set aside and keep warm.

2. Add the butter to the pot and melt over medium heat. Add the garlic and black pepper and sauté for 2 minutes. Add the reserved pasta water and stir well. Add the cheese and whisk until it melts and forms a thin sauce.

3. Add the pasta back to the pot and toss together until evenly coated. Top with more grated cheese and serve.

Serving Suggestion: Serve this dish with a light salad, and it also goes great with the Lemon and Herb Scallops (page 93). The peppery pasta and the light lemony scallops are a scrumptious match.

Easiest Baked Mac and Cheese

PREP TIME *15 MINUTES*   **COOK TIME** *45 MINUTES*   **SERVES** *6*

QUICK PREP   VEGETARIAN

Ditch the boxed macaroni and cheese and make this easy recipe at home. It's extra cheesy and requires only a few staple ingredients. Once you realize how simple and delicious this creamy macaroni and cheese recipe is, you will never go back to the box.

Main Ingredients

12 ounces elbow macaroni

2 tablespoons butter

⅓ cup all-purpose flour

3 cups 2 percent milk

1 pound sharp cheddar cheese, shredded, divided

Pantry Staples

Nonstick cooking spray

1 teaspoon salt

½ teaspoon black pepper

1. Preheat the oven to 350°F. Coat a casserole dish with cooking spray.

2. Bring a large pot of water to a boil over high heat. Add the macaroni and cook until al dente or according to the package instructions, 9 to 12 minutes. Drain well.

3. In the same pot, melt the butter over medium heat. Add the flour and, while whisking, slowly add the milk. Lower the heat to low and cook until thickened, 4 to 5 minutes.

4. Add the salt, the black pepper, and 12 ounces of shredded cheese and mix well until the cheese melts and the sauce is smooth. Add the pasta and mix until well combined and heated through.

5. Transfer the mixture into the prepared casserole dish and sprinkle with the remaining cheese.

6. Bake for about 25 minutes, or until the casserole is bubbling around the edges and the cheese on top is starting to brown. Let cool for a few minutes and serve.

Cooking Tip: This casserole can easily be made up to a day in advance and heated up when ready to serve. Wrap the casserole in plastic wrap after step 5 and when ready to heat, unwrap and place in a 350°F oven for 25 to 30 minutes, or until bubbling.

Penne with Broccoli Pesto

PREP TIME *5 MINUTES*   **COOK TIME** *25 MINUTES*   **SERVES** *6*

30 MINUTES OR LESS   QUICK PREP   VEGETARIAN

The ingredients of this mouthwatering pesto sauce might surprise your family, as the main ingredient is broccoli. To create the pesto, the broccoli is cooked down until it turns into a sauce that will coat the pasta. It's combined with garlic, lemon, and Parmesan to create a delicious pesto sauce.

Main Ingredients

1 (16-ounce) package penne pasta

4 garlic cloves, crushed

1 pound frozen broccoli

Juice of 1 lemon

½ cup grated vegetarian Parmesan cheese, plus extra for serving

Pantry ingredients

Salt and black pepper   ¼ cup olive oil

1. Bring a large pot of salted water to a boil over medium-high heat. Add the pasta and cook until almost al dente, about 8 minutes. Reserve ¾ cup of the pasta water and drain the pasta.

2. While the pasta is cooking, heat the olive oil in a large skillet over medium heat. Add the garlic and sauté until it starts to brown, about 2 minutes. Add the broccoli and mix well to coat evenly with the oil. Add the lemon juice and cook until the broccoli starts to fall apart, about 10 minutes. Add the reserved pasta water and mix thoroughly to form a sauce. There will still be some broccoli pieces mixed in.

3. Transfer the pasta to the skillet, toss with the sauce until evenly coated, and cook until the sauce thickens.

4. Remove the pan from the heat, add the Parmesan cheese, and toss until combined. Season well with salt and black pepper. Top with extra grated cheese if desired and serve.

Serving Suggestion: While this pasta dish is great by itself, it makes a nice side for most poultry or beef dishes, including grilled steak or roasted chicken.

Shrimp Orzo Skillet

PREP TIME 15 MINUTES   **COOK TIME 25 MINUTES**   **SERVES 4**

DAIRY-FREE   QUICK PREP

This shrimp and orzo recipe contains only a few simple ingredients and is packed with flavor from the tomatoes and herbs. Peas offer a contrasting color and add fiber to the recipe. Keep in mind that shrimp cook very quickly, so make sure not to overcook them in this dish.

Main Ingredients

1 (12-ounce) package orzo pasta (or another small pasta like ditalini)

1 (14-ounce) can diced tomatoes with garlic and onion

2 cups frozen peas

12 ounces large shrimp, peeled and deveined

3 tablespoons chopped fresh basil

Pantry Ingredients

2 tablespoons olive oil

Salt and black pepper

1. Bring a large pot of water to a boil over medium-high heat. Add the orzo and cook until al dente, about 6 minutes. Reserve ½ cup of the pasta water and drain the orzo.

2. While the pasta is cooking, heat the oil in a large skillet over medium heat. Add the tomatoes and peas and cook, stirring occasionally, until the peas are no longer frozen, about 10 minutes. Add the shrimp and cook until they start to turn pink, about 5 minutes.

3. Lower the heat to low, add the orzo and reserved pasta water, and cook until everything is heated through and the sauce thickens, 3 to 4 minutes. Add the basil and toss with the pasta until the basil is slightly wilted.

4. Season with salt and black pepper to taste and serve.

Substitution Tip: For a variation, drain and rinse 1 (14-ounce) can artichoke hearts and roughly chop them. Substitute the artichokes for the frozen peas.

Easy Baked Ziti Casserole

PREP TIME *15 MINUTES*   **COOK TIME** *1 HOUR 5 MINUTES*   **SERVES** *6*

QUICK PREP

This classic pasta bake is made with a tomato-based meat sauce and topped with a generous amount of cheese. The result is a hot and bubbly casserole full of hearty goodness coming out of the oven!

Main Ingredients

1 (16-ounce) package ziti or rigatoni pasta

1 pound ground beef

1 (28- or 32-ounce) jar marinara sauce

2 cups ricotta cheese

12 ounces shredded Italian blend cheese, divided

Pantry Staples

Nonstick cooking spray

1 tablespoon olive oil

1. Preheat the oven to 350°F. Coat a large casserole dish with cooking spray.

2. Bring a large pot of water to a boil over medium-high heat. Add the pasta and cook until al dente, according to the package instructions, 9 to 12 minutes for ziti, 10 to 14 minutes for rigatoni. Drain the pasta, set aside, and keep warm.

3. In a large skillet over medium-high heat, heat the olive oil. Add the ground beef and cook, breaking up the meat with a spoon, until browned and no longer pink, about 10 minutes. Drain any excess grease. Lower the heat to low, add the marinara sauce, and simmer, stirring occasionally, until the sauce thickens, about 10 minutes.

4. In a large bowl, toss together the drained pasta and meat sauce until evenly coated. Add the ricotta cheese and all but 1 cup of the Italian blend cheese and stir until combined. Transfer the pasta mixture to the prepared casserole dish and sprinkle with the remaining 1 cup of Italian cheese blend.

5. Loosely cover the dish with foil and bake for 20 minutes. Remove the foil and bake for another 10 minutes until the cheese on top is bubbly. Serve hot.

Leftover Tip: This casserole will leave you with leftovers and is easy to reheat in individual portions. Just cover the plate with a loose paper towel and microwave for 60 to 90 seconds. Continue to microwave in 15-second increments until heated through.

Penne Florentine with Bacon

PREP TIME 10 MINUTES   **COOK TIME** 30 MINUTES   **SERVES** 6

ONE POT   QUICK PREP   DAIRY-FREE

Although "Florentine" in cooking traditionally means that the food originates from Florence, Italy, and is plated on a bed of spinach, it has come to mean any Italian-style dish that features spinach. For this recipe, you can add the leafy green to the pasta to increase the nutritional value of the meal and add a vegetable to your kiddos' diet. Bacon adds extra flavor to the recipe!

Main Ingredients

1 (16-ounce) package penne pasta

3 garlic cloves, minced

1 (10-ounce) package frozen spinach, defrosted

1 cup chicken broth, or more if needed

4 ounces cooked bacon, crumbled

Pantry Staples

2 tablespoons olive oil

Salt and black pepper

1. Bring a large pot of water to a boil over medium-high heat. Add the pasta and cook until al dente, according to the package instructions, 10 to 13 minutes. Drain the pasta and set aside to keep warm.

2. In the same pot, heat the olive oil over medium-high heat. Add the garlic and cook until softened, 2 to 3 minutes.

3. Add the spinach, stir well, and cook until bubbly, about 10 minutes.

4. Lower the heat to low, add the penne and broth, and cook until the sauce is well blended and thickened. Add extra broth if needed to reach your desired consistency. Add the bacon and toss with the pasta right before serving.

5. Transfer the pasta into a large bowl, season with salt and black pepper to taste, and serve.

Cooking Tip: Bacon can easily be prepared in the microwave. Place paper towels on a microwave-safe plate and lay bacon slices in a single layer on top. Place a few paper towels on top. Microwave for 2 to 3 minutes or until cooked to desired consistency.

Rigatoni with Sausage and Chunky Tomato Sauce

PREP TIME *10 MINUTES*   **COOK TIME** *45 MINUTES*   **SERVES** *6*

DAIRY-FREE   QUICK PREP

Delicious pieces of sausage are combined with a tomato-garlic sauce and rigatoni pasta for a quick and easy healthy meal option. It's definitely helpful to keep pasta and canned tomatoes on hand in your pantry to be able to quickly prepare a tomato-based pasta recipe.

Main Ingredients

1 (16-ounce) package rigatoni pasta

12 ounces bulk Italian sausage

3 garlic cloves, chopped

1 (28-ounce) can petite diced tomatoes

1 tablespoon dried Italian seasoning

Pantry Ingredients

1 tablespoon olive oil

Salt and black pepper

1. Bring a large pot of water to a boil over medium-high heat. Add the pasta and cook until al dente, according to the package instructions, for 10 to 14 minutes. Drain the pasta, set aside, and keep warm.

2. While the pasta is cooking, heat the olive oil in a large skillet over medium-high heat. Add the sausage and cook, breaking up the meat with a spoon, until cooked through and no longer pink, 5 to 7 minutes. Lower the heat to low, add the garlic, tomatoes, and Italian seasoning, and cook, stirring occasionally, for 20 minutes.

3. Add the pasta to the sauce, stir well, and cook until the pasta and sauce are well blended, another 3 or 4 minutes.

4. Season with salt and black pepper to taste and serve.

Cooking Tip: A lot of people prefer pasta cooked al dente or "to the tooth." For perfectly cooked pasta, when it gets close to the estimated cooking time, taste it and see if it is at the desired consistency. Remember, you can always cook it longer, but you can't uncook it!

Super Easy Chicken Fried Rice

PREP TIME *10 MINUTES*　　　**COOK TIME** *20 MINUTES*　　　**SERVES** *4*

30 MINUTES OR LESS　　**DAIRY-FREE**　　**GLUTEN-FREE**　　**ONE PAN**　　**QUICK PREP**

Homemade fried rice is a meal that is endlessly adaptable to what you have on hand. The recipe comes together so quickly and can be a delicious weeknight meal. Frozen mixed vegetables and packet rice make this recipe a breeze to cook.

Main Ingredients

2 boneless, skinless chicken thighs, cut into 1-inch pieces

1 (10-ounce) package frozen mixed vegetables

3 cups precooked rice, homemade or store bought

3 tablespoons gluten-free soy sauce, plus extra if needed

2 eggs, beaten

Pantry Staples

2 tablespoons olive oil

Salt and black pepper

1. In a large skillet over medium-high heat, heat the olive oil. Add the chicken thighs and cook until they start to brown and are no longer pink, about 5 minutes. Add the frozen vegetables and sauté until they are soft, about 5 minutes.

2. Add the rice and soy sauce and cook, stirring frequently, until the rice is fried, about 3 minutes.

3. Push the rice mixture to one side of the pan and add the eggs to the empty side. Stir well with a spoon or a spatula and cook until the eggs are scrambled. Mix the eggs with the fried rice until completely combined. Remove the pan from the heat.

4. Season with salt and black pepper or extra soy sauce if desired and serve.

Substitution Tip: If you feel like using a different protein, try 2 cups of small shelled shrimp, 6 ounces of ground pork, or 1½ cups of cubed tofu instead of the chicken. If you have leftover rice in your refrigerator, you can substitute that for packaged rice, but make sure it is cold when you add it to the pan.

Easiest Butternut Squash Risotto

PREP TIME *10 MINUTES*   **COOK TIME** *35 MINUTES*   **SERVES** *4*

GLUTEN-FREE   ONE PAN   QUICK PREP   VEGETARIAN

Few dishes can compare to a bowl of creamy risotto. It may seem like a fancy dish, but it is actually easy to make, and the combination of butternut squash and Parmesan cheese is a match made in heaven. Risotto is a hearty and filling treat on a cold and blustery day.

Main Ingredients

⅓ cup finely chopped onions

2 cups cubed butternut squash

1 cup arborio rice

2 to 3 cups low-sodium vegetable stock or broth, heated

½ cup grated vegetarian Parmesan cheese

Pantry Staples

2 tablespoons olive oil

Salt and black pepper

1. In a large skillet over medium-high heat, heat the olive oil. Add the onions and butternut squash and sauté until they start to soften, about 5 minutes.

2. Add the rice, lower the heat to medium, and cook until the rice begins to turn translucent, 3 or 4 minutes.

3. Add the broth, one ladle at a time, every 3 to 5 minutes, stirring occasionally to keep the rice from sticking to the pan, waiting until the liquid is absorbed by the rice before adding another ladle of broth. The risotto is done when the rice is creamy and tender, 20 to 25 minutes total.

4. Add the Parmesan cheese and stir until melted. Season with salt and black pepper to taste and serve.

Cooking Tip: Heat up the broth in a small pan and keep it simmering as you add it to the risotto.

California Veggie Barley Bowls

PREP TIME *10 MINUTES*   **COOK TIME** *30 MINUTES*   **SERVES** *4*

QUICK PREP   VEGAN

Grain and veggie bowls are trending on many restaurant menus lately, but they are a simple recipe you can create at home. Barley is a healthy grain with a slightly nutty chew that works perfectly with these veggies and beans. This vegan meal is perfect when you want a simple healthy recipe.

Main Ingredients

1 cup
quick-cooking barley

1 (12-ounce) bag frozen
California vegetable blend

1 (14-ounce) can pinto
beans, drained and rinsed

2 small avocados, pitted,
peeled, and diced

1 cup salsa

Pantry Staples

2 tablespoons olive
oil, divided

Salt and black pepper

1. In a medium saucepan, cook the barley according to the package instructions, about 15 minutes.

2. In a large skillet over medium-high heat, mix together the frozen vegetables and 1 tablespoon of olive oil. Cook until the vegetables are heated through, about 7 minutes. Transfer the vegetables to a bowl and set aside.

3. Lower the heat to medium, add the beans and the remaining 1 tablespoon of olive oil to the same skillet, and cook until heated through, about 5 minutes.

4. To assemble the bowls, spoon an equal amount of barley, vegetables, beans, and diced avocado into each bowl. Season with salt and black pepper. Serve warm or at room temperature. Top with the salsa or serve it on the side.

Substitution Tip: A California vegetable blend usually includes carrots, broccoli, and cauliflower. To make this bowl a bit different, try a Southwest vegetable blend or really any veggie blend that you like.

Farro with Zucchini and Walnuts

PREP TIME *10 MINUTES*   **COOK TIME** *15 MINUTES*   **SERVES** *4*
PLUS 30 MINUTES RESTING TIME

QUICK PREP   VEGETARIAN

This nutrition-packed dish can be served as either a main or a side, but with ingredients like whole grains, cheese, and nuts, it definitely feels like a complete meal. While cooking the farro takes some time, even that step is simple. Once the salad is made, it keeps well for several days, so making it ahead can also make things easier.

Main Ingredients

1½ cups farro

¼ cup red wine vinegar

3 medium zucchini, cut into ¼-inch-thick half-moon

½ cup shaved vegetarian Parmesan cheese

¾ cup walnut halves or pieces

Pantry Staples

Salt and black pepper

¼ cup olive oil

1. In a medium saucepan, combine the farro, a pinch of salt, and enough water to cover by 2 to 3 inches. Bring to a boil over high heat and cook until the grains are tender, about 15 minutes. Strain, then let cool briefly.

2. While the farro is cooking, prepare the dressing. In a small mixing bowl, whisk the olive oil and red wine vinegar. Add salt and pepper to taste and whisk until combined.

3. Reserve 1 to 2 tablespoons each of Parmesan cheese and walnuts to sprinkle on top of the salad. In a medium mixing bowl, combine the farro, zucchini, remaining walnuts, and remaining Parmesan cheese. Pour the dressing over the farro mixture and stir until coated. Cover, transfer the bowl to the refrigerator, and let rest for at least 30 minutes to allow the dressing flavors to develop.

4. When ready to serve, remove from the fridge and garnish with the reserved Parmesan cheese and walnuts.

Leftover Tip: Store leftover salad in an airtight container in the fridge for up to 4 days.

Ingredient Tip: To make this an even more satiating meal, add a can of drained chickpeas and double the amount of dressing, or top with canned fish such as tuna or salmon.

Couscous with Lemon Chicken and Olives

PREP TIME *10 MINUTES*   **COOK TIME** *20 MINUTES*   **SERVES** *6*

30 MINUTES OR LESS   DAIRY-FREE   ONE PAN   QUICK PREP

The contrasting ingredients in this simple recipe pack a super flavorful punch! Couscous is made from durum wheat and looks like very tiny pasta. Because it is so small, it cooks up quickly, making it a very convenient ingredient. It has a nutty taste and will take on any flavors you cook with it.

Main Ingredients

1 pound boneless, skinless chicken thighs, cut into bite-size pieces

Zest and juice of 1 lemon

1 cup pitted green olives, cut in half

1 (10-ounce) package couscous

3 tablespoons chopped fresh parsley

Pantry Staples

1 to 2 tablespoons olive oil   Salt and black pepper

1. In a large skillet with a lid over medium-high heat, heat the olive oil. Add the chicken and cook until cooked through and lightly browned, about 10 minutes. Season with salt and black pepper.

2. Sprinkle the lemon zest and lemon juice over the chicken. Add the olives and cook, stirring occasionally, for another 3 minutes.

3. Pour in 4 cups of water and bring to a boil. Stir in the couscous, cover the pan, turn off the heat, and let stand for 5 minutes. Mix in the parsley, fluff with a fork, and season with more salt and black pepper, if desired. Serve warm.

Serving Suggestion: Serve Garlicky Peas and Mushrooms (page 116) on the side to make this a complete meal.

Quinoa with Spicy Black Beans and Sausage

PREP TIME *10 MINUTES*   **COOK TIME** *35 MINUTES*   **SERVES** *4*

DAIRY-FREE   **GLUTEN-FREE**   **QUICK PREP**

If you are looking for a healthier base for your bowls, then quinoa is for you. You can use a spicy chicken sausage along with fire-roasted tomatoes and chili powder to give this dish some heat. If you don't like your food that spicy, you can use any type of sausage and a can of plain diced tomatoes to create a less-spicy version of the recipe.

Main Ingredients

1 cup quinoa

12 ounces spicy smoked turkey sausage or chicken sausage, cut into bite-size pieces

1 (15-ounce) can black beans, drained and rinsed

1 (14-ounce) can diced fire-roasted tomatoes

1 tablespoon chili powder

Pantry Ingredients

1 tablespoon olive oil

1. Rinse the quinoa in a colander with cold water. In a medium saucepan over medium-high heat, combine the quinoa and 2 cups of water. Cook until the mixture comes to a rolling boil. Lower the heat to low and simmer until the quinoa is tender but not mushy and the water has been absorbed, 10 to 15 minutes. Remove from the heat and fluff with a fork.

2. In a large skillet over medium-high heat, heat the olive oil. Add the sausage and cook until it starts to brown, about 5 minutes. Add the black beans, tomatoes, and chili powder and stir well. Bring the mixture to a simmer, cover, lower the heat to low, and cook for 10 more minutes.

3. Combine the quinoa with the sausage and bean mixture. Spoon into bowls and serve.

Ingredient tip: Quinoa needs to be rinsed to remove its natural coating and take away any bitterness. You can also buy prerinsed quinoa that will save you a step.

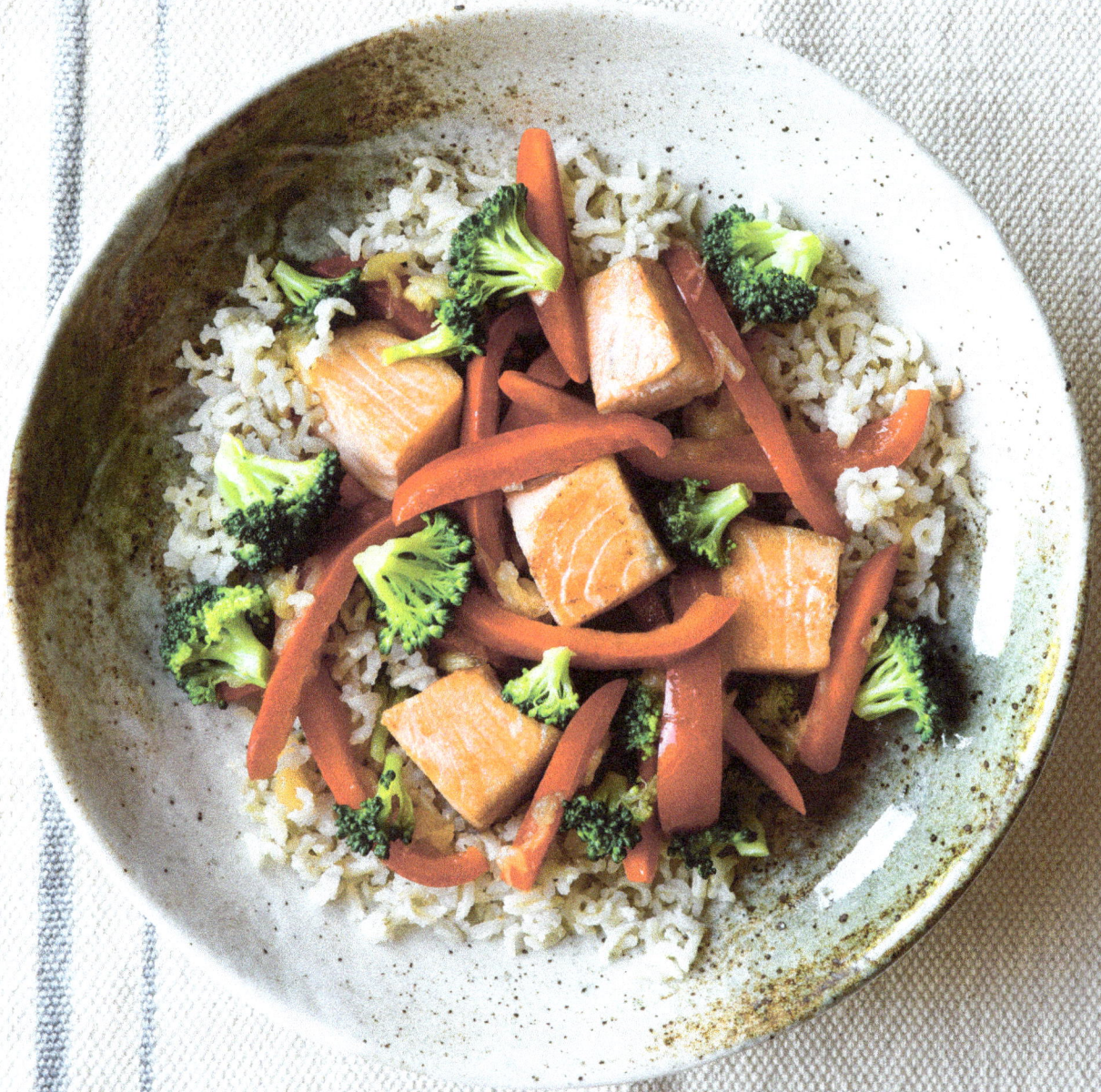

SHEET PAN LEMON-GARLIC SALMON AND VEGGIE BOWL · 88

Chapter Five
MEAT AND SEAFOOD MEALS

66 **Lemon Oregano Chicken Skewers with Yogurt Sauce**

67 **Chicken Enchiladas Verde**

68 **Chicken Milanese with Arugula**

69 **Baked Chicken Thighs with Tomatoes and Feta**

70 **Sunday Roast Chicken Dinner**

71 **Roasted BBQ Turkey Drumsticks**

72 **Turkey Cutlets with White Wine and Mushrooms**

74 **Ground Beef and String Bean Stir-Fry**

75 **French Onion Burgers**

76 **Pan-Seared Sirloin Tips with Mushrooms**

77 **Soy-Marinated Flank Steak**

78 **Chili-Rubbed Steak and Red Pepper Kebabs**

79 **Peppery Chicken-Fried Cube Steaks**

80 **The Ultimate Philly Cheesesteak**

81 **Red Gravy Pot Roast**

82 **Sheet Pan Sausage, Poblano Pepper, and Potatoes**

83 **Hawaiian Pork and Pineapple Kebabs**

84 **Open-Faced Pulled Pork Sandwiches**

85 **Pork Chop Fajita Skillet**

86 **Lemon Pepper Pork Tenderloin with Roasted Root Vegetables**

88 **Sheet Pan Lemon-Garlic Salmon and Veggie Bowl**

89 **Lemon-Dill Salmon Packet**

90 **Sheet Pan Baked Fish and Chips**

91 **Seared Tuna Steaks with Slaw**

92 **Shrimp and Avocado Tostadas**

93 **Lemon and Herb Scallops**

Lemon Oregano Chicken Skewers with Yogurt Sauce

PREP TIME 15 MINUTES   COOK TIME 25 MINUTES

MARINATING TIME 30 MINUTES   SERVES 4

GLUTEN-FREE ONE PAN

Surprisingly, Greek yogurt can be added to many savory recipes such as these chicken skewers. The creamy sauce goes great with the bold flavors of lemon and oregano.

Main Ingredients

1 cup plain Greek yogurt

Juice of 2 lemons, divided

1 pound boneless, skinless chicken breasts, cut into 1- to 2-inch cubes

1 tablespoon dried oregano

3 garlic cloves, minced

Pantry Staples

Salt and black pepper

2 tablespoons olive oil

1. In a small bowl, mix together the yogurt and half the lemon juice. Season with salt and black pepper. Cover and refrigerate the sauce until ready to serve.

2. In a medium bowl, mix together the chicken, oregano, garlic, olive oil, ½ teaspoon salt, and the remaining lemon juice. Add the chicken, cover, and refrigerate for at least 30 minutes or up to 8 hours.

3. Preheat oven to 400°F. Line a sheet pan with parchment paper or spray it with cooking spray.

4. Thread the chicken tightly onto 4 wooden or metal skewers. Discard any left-over marinade.

5. Place the skewers on the sheet pan and bake for 10 minutes. Turn the skewers over and bake for another 10 to 15 minutes, or until the chicken is no longer pink and the juices run clear. Serve the skewers with the yogurt sauce on the side.

Cooking Tip: If you are using wooden skewers, soak them in water for a few hours before threading them with the chicken. This will keep them from burning while the chicken is cooking.

Chicken Enchiladas Verde

PREP TIME *20 MINUTES* **COOK TIME** *25 MINUTES* **SERVES** *4*

GLUTEN-FREE ONE PAN

The thought of making homemade enchiladas can definitely seem overwhelming if you have never done it. This recipe keeps the ingredient list straightforward and the preparation nearly effortless with a tangy store-bought salsa verde and a generous amount of white cheddar cheese!

Main Ingredients

3 cups shredded cooked chicken

2 cups salsa verde, divided

3 cups shredded white cheddar cheese, divided

½ cup sour cream, plus extra for serving

8 corn tortillas, warmed

Pantry Staples

Nonstick cooking spray

1. Preheat the oven to 350°F. Spray a baking dish or casserole with cooking spray.

2. In a medium bowl, mix together the chicken, ½ cup of salsa verde, and 2 cups of cheese.

3. In another medium bowl, mix together the remaining 1½ cups of salsa verde and the sour cream. Spoon some of the sauce into the prepared baking dish and lightly coat the bottom.

4. Fill the tortillas with the chicken mixture, roll them up, and place them in the prepared pan, seam-side down.

5. Pour the remaining salsa verde sauce over the enchiladas and sprinkle with the remaining 1 cup of cheese. Bake for 25 minutes, or until the cheese is bubbling. Serve hot with extra sour cream, if desired.

Cooking Tip: To make the corn tortillas easier to work with, wrap a stack of tortillas in damp paper towels and place them in a microwave-safe dish. Microwave for 15 to 20 seconds or until they are warm and pliable.

Chicken Milanese with Arugula

PREP TIME *15 MINUTES*   **COOK TIME** *20 MINUTES*   **SERVES** *4*

DAIRY-FREE   ONE PAN   QUICK PREP

Chicken Milanese is a simple Italian dish of thin cutlets that are coated with bread crumbs and quickly sautéed. You can serve it on a bed of peppery arugula flavored with lemon to add extra flavor and a vegetable source.

Main Ingredients

1 large egg

⅔ cup Italian-seasoned panko bread crumbs

1 pound thin-cut chicken cutlets

6 ounces arugula

Juice of 1 lemon

Pantry Staples

¼ cup plus 2 tablespoons olive oil, divided

Salt and black pepper

1. In a shallow bowl, beat together the egg and 2 tablespoons of water and set aside. Put the bread crumbs in another shallow bowl.

2. Dip each chicken cutlet first into the egg mixture and then into the bread crumbs until they are evenly coated on both sides. Set them aside on a plate.

3. In a large skillet over medium heat, heat ¼ cup of olive oil. Add the chicken cutlets to the pan and cook until the chicken is golden brown and no longer pink inside, 4 to 6 minutes on each side. Transfer the chicken to a plate and set aside.

4. In a medium bowl, toss together the arugula, the lemon juice, and the remaining 2 tablespoons of olive oil. Season with salt and black pepper to taste.

5. Place the chicken cutlets on top of the dressed arugula and serve.

Cooking Tip: Thin-cut chicken cutlets work best in this recipe and can be purchased prepackaged at most grocery stores. If you can't find them or want to save money by purchasing a big pack of chicken breasts, you can easily make them thinner yourself. Place the boneless chicken breasts between two pieces of waxed paper or plastic wrap or in a resealable plastic bag. Starting with the center and working out to the edges, pound the chicken breasts lightly with the flat side of a meat mallet until the chicken is the desired thickness.

Baked Chicken Thighs with Tomatoes and Feta

PREP TIME *10 MINUTES*   **COOK TIME** *50 MINUTES*   **SERVES** *4*

GLUTEN-FREE   QUICK PREP

Keeping chicken in the freezer is a great shortcut to dinner any night. This delicious recipe combines salty, flavorful feta cheese with tangy cherry tomatoes for a creamy, flavorful topping to add to chicken thighs. Garlic and chicken broth add additional flavor to this recipe.

Main Ingredients

8 bone-in, skin-on chicken thighs

3 garlic cloves, minced

1 pint cherry tomatoes, halved

1 cup chicken broth

½ cup feta cheese

Pantry Staples

Salt and black pepper

2 tablespoons olive oil

1. Preheat the oven to 375°F.

2. Sprinkle the salt and black pepper on both sides of the chicken thighs.

3. In a large skillet over medium-high heat, heat the olive oil. Add the chicken thighs and cook until they start to brown, about 5 minutes on each side. Cook in batches if all the chicken cannot fit in one pan. Transfer the chicken to a baking dish or roasting pan.

4. Add the garlic, tomatoes, and broth to the skillet and cook until the tomatoes wilt and the mixture comes to a boil, about 5 minutes. Season with salt and black pepper to taste.

5. Pour the tomato mixture evenly over the chicken in the baking dish. Bake for 35 minutes, or until the chicken is cooked through and the internal temperature is 165°F. If you would like crispier skin, you can turn the oven to broil for the last few minutes of cooking.

6. Transfer the chicken and tomato mixture to a platter, sprinkle with feta cheese, and serve.

Sunday Roast Chicken Dinner

PREP TIME *15 MINUTES*   **COOK TIME** *40 MINUTES*   **SERVES** *4*

DAIRY-FREE   **GLUTEN-FREE**   **ONE PAN**   **QUICK PREP**

A few pantry staples and minimal preparation result in a roasted chicken full of tenderness and flavor. One of the best things about having a roasted chicken for dinner is the intoxicating aroma in the kitchen while it is cooking. Leftovers are always an added bonus when preparing chicken recipes! The leftovers can be reinvented into another chicken recipe for lunch or dinner the next day.

Main Ingredients

1 (3- or 4-pound) roasting chicken, cut into 8 pieces

1 to 2 tablespoons dried rosemary

1½ pounds baby potatoes

2 large carrots, cut into 2-inch pieces

2 medium onions, peeled and quartered

Pantry Staples

2 tablespoons olive oil, divided

Salt and pepper

1. Preheat the oven to 400°F.

2. Trim any excess fat from the chicken and pat it dry with paper towels. Rub 1 tablespoon of olive oil all over the chicken pieces and season them with salt, pepper, and 1 tablespoon of rosemary. Add more rosemary if desired.

3. In a bowl, toss together the potatoes, carrots, onions, salt, and pepper and the remaining 1 tablespoon of olive oil. Spread the vegetables and the chicken on a large, rimmed sheet pan.

4. Roast for 30 to 40 minutes, until the juices run clear or until a meat thermometer placed in the thickest chicken piece reaches 165°F.

5. Transfer the chicken and vegetables to a platter, let rest for a few minutes, and serve.

Leftover Tip: The leftover chicken is great to use in soups, salads, or sandwiches. You can use it for the Chicken Enchiladas Verde (page 67).

Roasted BBQ Turkey Drumsticks

PREP TIME *10 MINUTES*   **COOK TIME** *1 HOUR 25 MINUTES*   **SERVES** *4*

DAIRY-FREE   GLUTEN-FREE   ONE PAN   QUICK PREP

You may have seen the giant turkey legs people carry around and eat at amusement parks or festivals. You can also make these at home with only a few ingredients including barbecue seasoning and broth. The preparation for this recipe is effortless, but you will need some patience while these large pieces of poultry cook. The wait will be worth it!

Main Ingredients

4 medium turkey drumsticks

1 to 2 tablespoons barbecue seasoning or rub

½ cup low-sodium chicken broth

½ cup barbecue sauce, plus extra for serving

1. Preheat the oven to 350°F.

2. Pat the turkey legs dry with paper towels and place them on a large sheet pan or roasting pan. Rub the barbecue seasoning onto the drumsticks, making sure to get some under the skin.

3. Pour the chicken broth into the pan around the turkey legs.

4. Roast for 80 minutes, or until a meat thermometer placed in the thickest part of the drumstick registers 165°F.

5. Set the oven on broil.

6. Brush the barbecue sauce on the turkey legs, place the sheet pan back in the oven, and broil for 5 minutes.

7. Let the turkey legs cool for 10 minutes and serve.

Serving Suggestion: Serve these with Baked Sweet Potatoes with Cinnamon Honey (page 108). If you want a lower-carb side, serve with Cheesy Roasted Cauliflower (page 110) or Summer Squash Marinara (page 112).

Turkey Cutlets with White Wine and Mushrooms

PREP TIME 5 MINUTES   **COOK TIME 25 MINUTES**   **SERVES 4**

30 MINUTES OR LESS   **DAIRY-FREE**   **ONE PAN**   **QUICK PREP**

Your family might feel like they are turning into a chicken because they eat it so much! Change it up and try turkey cutlets instead. Topped with ample herbs, mushrooms, and white wine, they will banish any memory of dry Thanksgiving birds!

Main Ingredients

1 pound thin-cut turkey cutlets

⅓ cup all-purpose flour

1 cup white wine

10 ounces white mushrooms, sliced

2 tablespoons chopped fresh herbs, such as parsley or thyme

Pantry Staples

Salt and black pepper

2 tablespoons olive oil, plus extra if needed

1. Sprinkle the turkey cutlets with salt and black pepper on both sides. Lightly dip in the flour. Set aside on a plate.

2. In a large skillet over medium-high heat, heat the olive oil. Add the turkey cutlets and cook until the turkey is no longer pink, about 5 minutes on each side. If all the cutlets do not fit, cook them in two batches. You will need to add another 2 tablespoons of olive oil to the pan for the second batch. Transfer the turkey cutlets to a plate and cover them with aluminum foil to keep warm.

3. Add the wine to the skillet and deglaze the pan by using a spoon to scrape up all the brown bits from the bottom. When the liquid starts to simmer, lower the heat to medium, add the mushrooms, and cook until they are softened, about 6 minutes. Add the herbs to the pan.

4. Return the turkey to the pan. Spoon some of the sauce over the turkey, cover the pan, and lower the heat to low. It is okay if the pan is a little crowded at this point. Cook until the juices run clear and a meat thermometer inserted into the cutlet registers 165°F, about 5 minutes.

5. Season with salt and black pepper, transfer the cutlets to a serving plate, and spoon the sauce and mushrooms over the top. Serve hot.

Serving Suggestion: This turkey entrée goes perfectly with most of the side dishes in chapter 6. An excellent pairing is the Garlic Roasted Potatoes with Rosemary (page 109).

Ground Beef and String Bean Stir-Fry

PREP TIME *5 MINUTES*   COOK TIME *20 MINUTES*   SERVES *4*

30 MINUTES OR LESS   **DAIRY-FREE**   **ONE PAN**   **QUICK PREP**

Ground beef combines well with string beans. And it only gets better when served over a bowl of white or brown rice. If you would like a lower-carb meal, cauliflower rice is a really nice option. And you don't need to use green beans. Broccoli or a frozen stir-fry blend will also be great.

Main Ingredients

3 tablespoons barbecue sauce

2 tablespoons honey

2 tablespoons soy sauce

1 pound lean ground beef

1 pound frozen green beans

Pantry Staples

1 tablespoon olive oil

Salt and black pepper

1. In a small bowl, mix together the barbecue sauce, honey, and soy sauce. Set aside.

2. In a large skillet over high heat, heat the olive oil. Add the ground beef and sauté until it is cooked through and barely pink, about 5 minutes. Drain any extra grease if necessary.

3. Add the green beans and cook until they are cooked through, 5 to 10 minutes.

4. Pour the sauce into the skillet, mix well, and cook until the mixture is heated through.

5. Season with salt and black pepper to taste and serve.

Ingredient Tip: The barbecue sauce you use will really enhance the flavor of the dish, so if you like spicy food, be sure to use a spicy barbecue sauce. If you like it less sweet, be aware of the sugar content in the sauce you choose. You can also decrease the amount of honey in the recipe as another way to decrease the sweetness.

French Onion Burgers

PREP TIME *10 MINUTES*   COOK TIME *40 MINUTES*   SERVES *4*

ONE PAN   QUICK PREP

Most people feel inclined to cook their burgers on a grill, but there is nothing better than a big, juicy burger cooked inside on a skillet. It can be a time-saver not heating up the grill! These burgers have a great deal of flavor from the caramelized onions and melted cheese.

Main Ingredients

1 pound 80 percent lean ground beef

1 large onion, thinly sliced

¼ cup beef broth

4 thick slices Swiss cheese

4 hamburger buns

Pantry Staples

Salt and black pepper

2 tablespoons olive oil, divided

1. Form the ground beef into 4 equal patties. Season with salt and black pepper on both sides, place them on a plate, cover with plastic wrap, and refrigerate.

2. In a large skillet over medium-high heat, heat 1 tablespoon of olive oil. Add the onion and sauté until it starts to brown, about 5 minutes. Add the beef broth and use a wooden spoon to scrape any browned bits off the bottom of the pan. Lower the heat to low and cook, stirring occasionally, until the onion is caramelized, about 20 minutes Season with salt and black pepper. Transfer the onion to a bowl, cover, and keep warm.

3. Wipe out the skillet. Raise the heat to medium-high, add the remaining 1 tablespoon of olive oil, and cook the burgers for 5 minutes, flip them, and cook until the internal temperature reaches 160°F for well done, another 5 to 7 minutes. Cook less if desired for medium-rare.

4. Top the burgers with the cheese, cover the pan, and cook for 1 or 2 minutes until the cheese melts.

5. Place the burgers on buns, top with the caramelized onions and serve.

Serving Suggestion: Don't be shy with the toppings on your burger. Try pickles, ketchup, steak sauce, or any other condiments you like.

Pan-Seared Sirloin Tips with Mushrooms

PREP TIME *15 MINUTES*   **COOK TIME** *20 MINUTES*   **SERVES** *4*

DAIRY-FREE   GLUTEN-FREE   ONE PAN

There is nothing better than beef prepared with mushrooms and red wine! You don't need anything special—whatever you're drinking that night will do.

Main Ingredients

2 tablespoons steak seasoning

1 pound sirloin steak, cut in 1½-inch pieces

10 ounces white mushrooms, each cut in half

½ cup red wine

2 tablespoons chopped fresh parsley

Pantry Staples

1 tablespoon olive oil

Salt and black pepper

1. In a large bowl, toss the steak seasoning with the steak and mushrooms until evenly coated.

2. In a large skillet over medium-high heat, heat the olive oil.

3. Add the steak to the pan and cook, stirring occasionally, until it starts to brown, about 3 minutes. Transfer to a plate, cover, and keep warm.

4. Add the mushrooms to the skillet and cook, stirring occasionally, until they are softened and the juices are released, about 5 minutes. Add the wine to the pan, lower the heat to medium, and cook, stirring, until the liquid starts to reduce and the mushrooms are tender.

5. Return the steak to the pan and cook until it is cooked through but still a little pink on the inside or to your desired doneness, about 2 minutes.

6. Sprinkle with the parsley and season with salt and black pepper to taste.

Soy-Marinated Flank Steak

PREP TIME *10 MINUTES*

MARINATING TIME *1 HOUR*

COOK TIME *20 MINUTES*

SERVES *6*

DAIRY-FREE   ONE PAN

Flank steak is a lean but flavorful cut of meat. It is extremely tender when marinated and cut across the grain into slices. The marinade is filled with intense flavor and contributes a great deal to this melt-in-your-mouth main dish.

Main Ingredients

⅓ cup soy sauce

2 tablespoons maple syrup

3 garlic cloves, minced

3 scallions, thinly sliced, divided

2 pounds flank steak

Pantry Staples

2 tablespoons olive oil

1 tablespoon cider vinegar

½ teaspoon black pepper

1. In a medium bowl, mix together the soy sauce, maple syrup, garlic, olive oil, vinegar, and black pepper and 2 of the scallions.

2. Poke the steak all over with a fork and place it in a 1-gallon resealable plastic bag. Pour the marinade into the bag, remove as much air as possible, and seal. Place the steak flat in the refrigerator for at least 1 hour (or up to 12 hours), flipping it after 30 minutes so the steak marinates evenly.

3. Remove the steak from the marinade and discard the excess liquid. Pat the steak dry with paper towels and place it in a roasting pan.

4. Preheat the broiler.

5. Broil the steak until medium-rare, 7 to 8 minutes per side. Broil longer if you would like it more well done. Place the steak on a cutting board and let it sit for 5 minutes.

6. Cut the flank steak on an angle, against the grain, into thin slices.

7. Arrange on a platter and serve garnished with the remaining scallion.

Serving Suggestion: This steak goes particularly well with potatoes, so try it with the Garlic Roasted Potatoes with Rosemary (page 109).

Chili-Rubbed Steak and Red Pepper Kebabs

PREP TIME *20 MINUTES*

MARINATING TIME *2 HOURS*

COOK TIME *30 MINUTES*

SERVES *6*

DAIRY-FREE   GLUTEN-FREE   ONE PAN

With both meat and vegetables on each skewer, kabobs make a complete meal. If you have a grill, that's a great alternative cooking method—just be sure to soak your skewers so they don't burn.

Main Ingredients

1½ pounds sirloin steak, cut into 1- to 2-inch pieces

1 large onion, cut into 1- to 2-inch chunks

2 large bell peppers, cut into 1- to 2-inch chunks

8 to 10 ounces button mushrooms

2 tablespoons chili powder

Pantry Staples

2 tablespoons olive oil

Salt and black pepper

1. In a large bowl, mix together the steak, onion, bell peppers, mushrooms, and olive oil. Sprinkle the chili powder over the top and stir to evenly coat. Cover with plastic wrap and refrigerate for at least 2 hours and up to 8 hours.

2. Preheat the oven to 350°F.

3. Thread the meat and veggies onto metal skewers (or onto wooden skewers that have been soaked in water for 30 minutes), alternating the meat and vegetables.

4. Arrange the skewers on a large sheet pan and bake at 350°F for 30 minutes, or until the steak is cooked through, turning the skewers once.

5. Remove skewers from oven and let rest briefly. Season with salt and black pepper before serving.

Peppery Chicken-Fried Cube Steaks

PREP TIME *15 MINUTES*   **COOK TIME** *20 MINUTES*   **SERVES** *4*

ONE PAN   QUICK PREP

Despite its name, there is no chicken in this recipe! If you aren't familiar with cube steak, it's a less-expensive cut of beef that is pre-tenderized. It's most popularly used for chicken-fried steak recipes topped with a cream gravy. This recipe simplifies the traditional chicken-fried steak recipe by omitting the gravy but kicks up the flavor with lots of black pepper. It is delicious with Garlic Roasted Potatoes with Rosemary (page 109).

Main Ingredients

4 (4-ounce) cube steaks

⅓ cup all-purpose flour

¾ cup Italian-seasoned panko bread crumbs

1 large egg

2 tablespoons milk

Pantry Staples

Salt

1 teaspoon black pepper

About ½ cup olive oil

1. Preheat the oven to 250°F. Line a sheet pan with parchment paper or spray it with cooking spray.

2. Season the cube steaks with a sprinkle of salt. In a shallow bowl, combine the flour, bread crumbs, and black pepper. In a separate shallow bowl, beat together the egg and milk.

3. Dip the cube steaks into the bread crumb mixture and then the egg mixture. Dip them into the bread crumb mixture again until they are well coated. Place on a plate.

4. In a large skillet over medium-high heat, heat about 2 inches of oil. Carefully add the steaks to avoid spattering and cook, in batches if necessary, until golden brown, about 5 minutes on each side. Place the steaks on the prepared sheet pan and place in the oven to keep warm.

5. Serve hot.

Cooking Tip: The oil should be very hot when the steaks are added to the pan. To check, drop a little flour in the oil, and if little bubbles appear, it's ready.

The Ultimate Philly Cheesesteak

PREP TIME *10 MINUTES*   **COOK TIME** *25 MINUTES*   **SERVES** *4*

ONE PAN   QUICK PREP

If you have ever visited Philadelphia, chances are you've had a Philly cheesesteak. If you don't live in the area, it might be harder to find a Philly cheesesteak, but not to worry—you can prepare this delicious recipe at home with just a few easy ingredients including shaved chip steak, mushrooms, and onions.

Main Ingredients

1 large onion, thinly sliced

8 ounces mushrooms, sliced

1 pound shaved chip steak, roughly chopped

8 slices American cheese

4 (6-inch) hoagie rolls

Pantry Staples

2 tablespoons olive oil, divided

Salt and black pepper

1. In a large skillet over medium-high heat, heat 1 tablespoon of olive oil. Add the onion and mushrooms and cook until the onion starts to caramelize and the mushrooms are tender, 10 to 15 minutes. Transfer the vegetables to a bowl and keep warm.

2. Add the remaining 1 tablespoon of olive oil and the steak to the skillet and cook, stirring occasionally, until no longer pink, 5 to 10 minutes. Add the onion and mushrooms back to the pan and add salt and black pepper to taste. Top with the American cheese.

3. Lower the heat to low, cover the pan, and cook until the cheese is melted, about 30 seconds. Turn off the heat.

4. Split the hoagie rolls in half. Divide the meat mixture into four portions and, using a spatula, place each portion onto a roll.

5. Serve nice and hot.

Ingredient Tip: Chip steaks are superthin slices or shaved pieces of top round, typically sold in one-pound packages. If you cannot find it, thin-sliced sirloin or rib eye steak can be substituted.

Red Gravy Pot Roast

PREP TIME *10 MINUTES* **COOK TIME** *3 HOURS* **SERVES** *6*

DAIRY-FREE GLUTEN-FREE ONE POT QUICK PREP

If you have never tried a pot roast with red gravy rather than the more typical brown gravy, you must try this recipe. It takes a few hours to cook, but there is little prep work—you can quickly put it in the oven and then relax while your kitchen slowly fills with the delicious meaty aroma.

Main Ingredients

3 pounds beef bottom round roast

1 medium sweet onion, chopped

1 (28-ounce) can crushed tomatoes

3 garlic cloves, crushed

2 tablespoons Italian seasoning

Pantry Staples

Salt and black pepper

2 tablespoons olive oil

1. Preheat the oven to 325°F.

2. Season the roast with salt and black pepper.

3. In a large ovenproof pot with a lid or Dutch oven over medium-high heat, heat the olive oil. Add the roast and cook, turning the roast to brown on all sides, about 5 minutes. Add the onion and cook until it starts to turn translucent, about 5 minutes.

4. Add the tomatoes, garlic, Italian seasoning, and 1 cup of water and stir until combined. Bring the mixture to a boil, cover, and place the pot in the oven.

5. Bake for 2 to 2½ hours, or until the roast is fork-tender and the sauce has thickened. Add more water to thin out the sauce as needed.

6. Season with more salt and black pepper to taste. Cut the beef into thin slices and serve with extra sauce on the side.

Serving Suggestion: Serve the meat and gravy over pasta or rice. The thinly sliced pot roast is also great served as a sandwich on a hoagie roll.

Sheet Pan Sausage, Poblano Pepper, and Potatoes

PREP TIME *10 MINUTES*   **COOK TIME** *35 MINUTES*   **SERVES** *4*

DAIRY-FREE   **GLUTEN-FREE**   **ONE PAN**   **QUICK PREP**

Sheet pan dinners are great because everything cooks in one pan in the oven, leaving you time to get other things done. They also make for easy cleanup, especially if you line the sheet pan with parchment. This recipe also works nicely with any variety or flavor of sausage, including chicken or turkey.

Main Ingredients

1½ pounds baby potatoes, each cut in half

2 large poblano peppers, seeded and cut into slices

2 medium onions, peeled and quartered

2 teaspoons chili powder

1 pound pork sausage (about 5 links), cut into 2-inch pieces

Pantry Staples

1 tablespoon olive oil

½ teaspoon salt

1. Preheat the oven to 400°F. Line a large sheet pan with parchment paper or spray it with cooking spray.

2. In a large bowl, toss the potatoes, poblano peppers, onions, chili powder, olive oil, and salt until evenly coated.

3. Spread the vegetable mixture and sausage onto the sheet pan. Bake for 35 minutes, or until the potatoes are tender and the sausage is cooked through.

4. Serve hot.

Leftover Tip: Having leftovers from this recipe means you can chop it up the next day and quickly refry it in a pan for breakfast. Top it with fried or scrambled eggs to make a super delicious meal.

Hawaiian Pork and Pineapple Kebabs

PREP TIME *10 MINUTES*   **COOK TIME** *25 MINUTES*

MARINATING TIME *30 MINUTES*   **SERVES** *6*

DAIRY-FREE   **GLUTEN-FREE**   **ONE PAN**   **QUICK PREP**

Get a little taste of the tropics with these colorful and flavorful skewers. If you prefer chicken over pork, use cut-up chicken thighs—the kebabs are wonderful using either.

Main Ingredients

1½ pounds pork tenderloin, cut into 1- to 2-inch pieces

1 cup pineapple juice

2 red bell peppers, seeded and cut into 2-inch pieces

2 cups pineapple chunks

½ cup barbecue sauce, plus extra for serving

Pantry Staples

Salt and black pepper

1. In a medium bowl, season the pork with salt and black pepper. Add the pineapple juice, mix until combined, cover with plastic wrap, and refrigerate for 30 minutes to 1 hour.

2. Preheat the oven to 375°F. Line a sheet pan with parchment paper or spray it with cooking spray.

3. Thread the marinated pork, bell peppers, and pineapple onto metal or wooden skewers.

4. Arrange the skewers on the prepared sheet pan and brush them with the barbecue sauce.

5. Bake for 20 to 25 minutes, turning every 10 minutes, until the pork is cooked through. Turn the broiler on for the last few minutes of cooking to brown them a bit.

6. Serve hot.

Cooking Tip: If using wooden skewers, soak them in water for about 30 minutes before using so that they won't burn in the oven.

Open-Faced Pulled Pork Sandwiches

PREP TIME *10 MINUTES*   COOK TIME *1 HOUR 40 MINUTES*   SERVES *6*

DAIRY-FREE   ONE POT   QUICK PREP

Pulled pork is a great family meal that is easier to cook than most people think. You can use country-style boneless ribs in this recipe because they cook much quicker than a big roast.

Main Ingredients

1 medium onion, chopped

3 garlic cloves, minced

2 to 3 pounds boneless country-style pork ribs

1 cup barbecue sauce, plus more for serving

6 slices thick-cut sourdough or white bread, lightly toasted

Pantry Staples

1 tablespoon olive oil

1 teaspoon salt

½ teaspoon black pepper

1. In a large soup pot with a lid over medium-high heat, heat the olive oil. Add the onion and garlic and cook until golden, about 4 minutes. Place the pork in the pot and season it with salt and black pepper.

2. Pour the barbecue sauce and 1 cup of water over the meat and bring the mixture to a simmer. Lower the heat to low, cover the pot loosely, and cook until the meat is fork-tender and easily shreds, about 90 minutes.

3. Transfer the pork to a cutting board and shred it using a fork. Transfer the shredded pork to a large bowl, add some of the cooking liquid, and mix.

4. Spoon the pulled pork over the toasted bread slices and serve with extra barbecue sauce on the side.

Leftover Tip: This is a great recipe to make and keep in the freezer. Store it in an airtight container for up to 2 months. To reheat, defrost in the refrigerator overnight and then cook it in a saucepan for 10 to 15 minutes over medium heat, or until the sauce bubbles.

Pork Chop Fajita Skillet

PREP TIME *10 MINUTES*   **COOK TIME** *30 MINUTES*   **SERVES** *4*

DAIRY-FREE   **GLUTEN-FREE**   **ONE PAN**   **QUICK PREP**

These juicy pork chops are smothered with onions and peppers. The secret to perfectly cooked pork is to cook it to 145°F, and it's okay if it is still a little pink. It will be juicy and completely delicious. You can serve these chops with a side of warm tortillas for a complete dinner.

Main Ingredients

4 (6-ounce) bone-in pork chops

1 tablespoon chili powder

1 large onion, thinly sliced

2 red, yellow, or green bell peppers, seeded and cut into thin slices

Juice of 2 limes

Pantry Staples

2 tablespoons olive oil

Salt and black pepper

1. Sprinkle the pork chops with chili powder.

2. In a large skillet over medium-high heat, heat the olive oil. Add the chops and brown them on both sides, about 5 minutes per side. Transfer the pork chops to a plate and keep warm.

3. Lower the heat to medium, add the onion and bell peppers, and cook until just tender, about 5 minutes.

4. Stir in the lime juice and season with the salt and black pepper. Return the pork chops to the skillet and cover with the vegetables.

5. Lower the heat to low, cover, and simmer until the vegetables are soft, the chops are tender, and an instant-read meat thermometer reads 145°F, 10 to 15 minutes. Serve immediately.

Cooking Tip: An easy way to juice a lime is to first place it in the microwave oven for 20 seconds. This will release the juices and make it easy to get out the most liquid. Roll the lime on a cutting board and then cut it in half before juicing.

Lemon Pepper Pork Tenderloin with Roasted Root Vegetables

PREP TIME *10 MINUTES*   **COOK TIME** *40 MINUTES*   **SERVES** *6*

DAIRY-FREE   **GLUTEN-FREE**   **QUICK PREP**

Pork is the other white meat, and pork tenderloin is a lean cut that takes on the flavor of whatever seasoning you use. This hearty dinner seasoned with onions and lemon pepper is perfect on a chilly fall or winter night but can also be enjoyed during the hot summer months.

Main Ingredients

2 pounds Yukon Gold potatoes, cut into 1-inch cubes

3 cups baby carrots

2 medium onions, peeled and quartered

1½ to 2 pounds pork tenderloin

1 to 2 tablespoons lemon pepper seasoning

Pantry Staples

Salt and black pepper

2 tablespoons olive oil, divided

1. Preheat the oven to 400°F. Line a sheet pan with parchment paper or spray it with cooking spray.

2. In a large bowl, mix together the potatoes, carrots, and onions. Season with salt and black pepper. Drizzle the vegetables with 1 tablespoon of olive oil and toss together until well coated. Spread out the vegetables on the sheet pan in a single layer and roast for 20 minutes.

3. While the vegetables are cooking, in a medium bowl, toss the pork tenderloin with the remaining 1 tablespoon of olive oil and sprinkle with the lemon pepper seasoning, rubbing it in with your hands or a pastry brush, until the tenderloin is evenly coated.

4. In a large skillet over medium-high heat, sear the pork for 2 to 3 minutes on each side.

5. Once the vegetables have been baking for 20 minutes, use a spatula to turn them over. Place the pork tenderloin in the center of the sheet pan, pushing the vegetables to the sides. Return the sheet pan to the oven and roast for 15 to 20 minutes, or until an instant-read thermometer inserted in the pork reads 145°F for medium-rare or 160°F for medium.

6. Let the pork rest for 5 to 10 minutes before cutting it into slices. Place the slices on a platter along with the vegetables and serve.

Cooking Tip: To cut down on the preparation time for this recipe, you can purchase already marinated pork tenderloin and omit the seasoning. Most stores sell different types of flavors like lemon pepper, teriyaki, and barbecue, which all go well with the vegetables.

Sheet Pan Lemon-Garlic Salmon and Veggie Bowl

PREP TIME *10 MINUTES*   **COOK TIME** *25 MINUTES*   **SERVES** *4*

DAIRY-FREE   GLUTEN-FREE   ONE PAN   QUICK PREP

This healthy meal makes preparation and cleanup ridiculously easy by using just one sheet pan and roasting in the oven. The lemon-garlic marinade is punchy and delicious served over rice or other grains as well.

Main Ingredients

2 garlic cloves, minced

Juice from 1 to 2 lemons

3 cups fresh broccoli florets

1 red bell pepper, stemmed, seeded, and cut lengthwise into long, thin pieces

12 ounces skinless salmon fillets, cut into ¾-inch pieces

Pantry Staples

Nonstick cooking spray

⅓ cup olive oil

Salt and black pepper

1. Preheat the oven to 425°F. Spray a large sheet pan with nonstick cooking spray.

2. In a small bowl, whisk together the garlic, juice of 1 lemon, the olive oil, and a pinch of salt and pepper. Add more lemon juice, salt, and pepper to taste.

3. In a medium mixing bowl, combine the broccoli florets and red bell pepper, add 2 to 3 tablespoons of the marinade, and toss to ensure all the vegetables are well coated, adding more marinade as needed.

4. Spread the vegetables on the prepared sheet pan and bake for 10 to 15 minutes, or until lightly browned.

5. Remove the pan from the oven and add the salmon. Brush the remaining marinade over the salmon and vegetables and lightly season the salmon with salt and pepper. Return to the oven and bake for an additional 5 to 7 minutes, or until the salmon is opaque and cooked through. Divide the salmon and vegetables between four bowls and serve.

Lemon-Dill Salmon Packet

PREP TIME *10 MINUTES*   **COOK TIME** *15 MINUTES*   **SERVES** *4*

30 MINUTES OR LESS   DAIRY-FREE   GLUTEN-FREE   ONE PAN   QUICK PREP

Salmon is one of the easiest seafood choices to prepare. You can cook it a variety of ways, but one of the easiest options to create a juicy salmon piece is using foil packets. This recipe seasons the salmon with dill, garlic, and lemon for a bold and tart flavor.

Main Ingredients

1-pound salmon fillet, skin on

1 teaspoon garlic powder

1 tablespoon dried dill

1 large lemon, cut into thin slices

Pantry Staples

1 tablespoon olive oil

Salt and black pepper

1. Preheat the oven to 375°F. Place a large piece of aluminum foil on your work surface.

2. Rub both sides of the salmon with the olive oil and season it with salt, black pepper, and garlic powder. Place the salmon on the foil, skin-side down. Top with the dried dill and about ¾ of the lemon slices.

3. Fold the foil around the salmon to form a packet. Make sure the salmon is completely enclosed. Place the salmon on a sheet pan.

4. Bake for 15 minutes, or until the salmon is cooked completely and the internal temperature of the fish is 145°F. Carefully remove the salmon from the foil (watch out for steam), place it on a serving plate, and serve with extra lemon on the side, if desired.

Serving Suggestion: Serve on top of a bed of Wilted Balsamic Spinach (page 115).

Sheet Pan Baked Fish and Chips

PREP TIME *20 MINUTES*   **COOK TIME** *30 MINUTES*   **SERVES** *4*

DAIRY-FREE

Fish and chips are often a family favorite, but if you order them in a restaurant, they are deep fried. This lighter version can be made at home by baking the fish and potatoes in Italian-seasoned panko bread crumbs for a satisfying crunch that comes with less oil.

Main Ingredients

4 medium potatoes, scrubbed

2 cups Italian-seasoned panko bread crumbs

2 eggs, beaten

1 pound cod fillets, cut into 2- to 3-inch pieces

Pantry Staples

2 tablespoons olive oil

Salt and black pepper

Nonstick cooking spray

1. Preheat the oven to 425°F. Place an oven rack in the top position and one in the bottom position. Line 2 large sheet pans with parchment paper or spray them with cooking spray.

2. Cut the potatoes into ¼-inch sticks. Toss with the olive oil and sprinkle with ½ teaspoon of salt. Spread out the potatoes on one of the large sheet pans in a single layer and bake on the top rack for 15 minutes.

3. While the potatoes are baking, put the bread crumbs on a large plate and the eggs in a shallow bowl.

4. Season the fish with salt and black pepper. Dip the pieces into the egg mixture and then coat them with the bread crumbs, lightly pressing the crumbs onto the fish until they are well coated.

5. Place a wire rack on top of the second large sheet pan. Spray the rack with cooking spray. Place the fish on the rack.

6. After the potatoes have been baking for 15 minutes, flip them and return them to the top position in the oven. Place the sheet pan of fish on the bottom rack of the oven and bake for another 15 minutes, or until the fish is cooked through and both the fish and potatoes are crispy. Serve hot.

Seared Tuna Steaks with Slaw

PREP TIME *10 MINUTES*   **COOK TIME** *20 MINUTES*   **SERVES** *4*

30 MINUTES OR LESS   **DAIRY-FREE**   **ONE PAN**   **QUICK PREP**

Fresh tuna steaks can feel intimidating, but this simple tuna steak recipe can be prepared in less than 30 minutes and is topped with a delicious soy and sesame seed dressing.

Main Ingredients

1 tablespoon soy sauce

3 tablespoons sweet Asian chile sauce

6 cups coleslaw mix (8 to 10 ounces)

4 (4- to 6-ounce) tuna steaks

¼ cup black or white sesame seeds

Pantry Staples

4 tablespoons olive oil, divided

2 tablespoons cider vinegar

Salt and black pepper

1. In a small bowl, whisk together 3 tablespoons of olive oil, vinegar, soy sauce, and chile sauce. Reserve 2 tablespoons of the dressing and mix the remaining dressing in a large bowl with the coleslaw mix. Cover the bowl with plastic wrap and refrigerate until ready to use.

2. Rub the tuna with the remaining 1 tablespoon of olive oil and season with salt and black pepper. Press the sesame seeds onto the tuna until evenly coated.

3. Heat a large grill pan or skillet over medium-high heat. Sear the tuna until medium-rare, 3 to 4 minutes on each side. For more well done, cook for an additional 1 to 2 minutes per side.

4. Transfer the tuna to a plate and let rest for several minutes before cutting into slices. Drizzle the remaining dressing on top of the tuna.

5. Serve the tuna on top of the dressed coleslaw.

Leftover Tip: The leftovers from this tuna recipe can be used in tacos or wraps. To reheat, sear the tuna quickly in a nonstick pan and put it in a taco shell or tortilla wrap topped with the slaw mix. This might even be better than the original dinner!

Shrimp and Avocado Tostadas

PREP TIME *15 MINUTES*   **COOK TIME** *15 MINUTES*   **SERVES** *4*

30 MINUTES OR LESS   GLUTEN-FREE   QUICK PREP

Your themed meal for Tuesdays doesn't have to be just tacos. Mix it up a little with tostadas, which are like tacos but have a crispy flat shell, and they look beautiful on a plate. Shrimp and avocado are a delicious combination. The chunky salsa in this dish gives the shrimp tostadas a bold flavor.

Main Ingredients

8 taco-size soft flour tortillas

1 pound large shrimp, peeled and deveined

Juice of 1 lime

2 avocados, pitted, peeled, and mashed

1 cup chunky salsa

Pantry Staples

Olive oil

Salt and black pepper

1. In a medium nonstick skillet over medium-high heat, heat about ¼ inch of olive oil. One at a time, fry the tortillas until golden brown, about 30 seconds on each side. Remove from the pan and set aside on paper towels.

2. In a large skillet over medium-high heat, heat 2 tablespoons of olive oil. Add the shrimp and lime juice and cook, stirring occasionally, until the shrimp are pink and cooked through, 4 to 5 minutes. Season with salt and black pepper.

3. Spread the mashed avocado mixture on the tostadas. Top each with the shrimp and salsa and serve.

Ingredient Tip: To cut the preparation to only 5 minutes, buy shelled and deveined shrimp.

Lemon and Herb Scallops

PREP TIME *10 MINUTES*   **COOK TIME** *15 MINUTES*   **SERVES** *4*

30 MINUTES OR LESS   GLUTEN-FREE   ONE PAN   QUICK PREP

Scallops offer a light dish that is perfect for an elegant dinner. The buttery herb-lemon sauce is what takes this simple recipe from good to really great. For a full meal, serve it with steamed asparagus and slices of bread to sop up the sauce.

Main Ingredients

1 pound large scallops

2 to 3 tablespoons butter

Juice of 1 lemon plus 1 lemon cut into slices, for garnish

2 tablespoons chopped fresh herbs, such as parsley or tarragon, plus extra for garnish

Pantry Staples

1 tablespoon olive oil, plus more if needed

Salt and black pepper

1. Pat the scallops dry with paper towels. In a large skillet over medium-high heat, heat 2 tablespoons of olive oil.

2. Season the scallops with salt and black pepper. Add the scallops to the skillet in a single layer and cook, flipping once, until golden brown and translucent in the center, 1 to 2 minutes per side. If all the scallops do not fit, cook them in two batches. You will need to add another tablespoon of olive oil to the pan for the second batch. Transfer the scallops to a plate and keep warm.

3. Add the butter to the skillet and stir until melted. Stir in the lemon juice and chopped herbs. Season the sauce with salt and black pepper to taste.

4. Serve the scallops immediately with drizzles of the lemon butter sauce and garnished with herbs and lemon slices.

Ingredient Tip: Use your favorite fresh herbs or whatever you have on hand. You can use parsley, basil, tarragon, and sage in this recipe. They all give a unique freshness to this wonderful dish.

Serving Suggestion: You can serve these scallops on a bed of the Easiest Butternut Squash Risotto (page 58). They are also good with a side of rice or mashed potatoes.

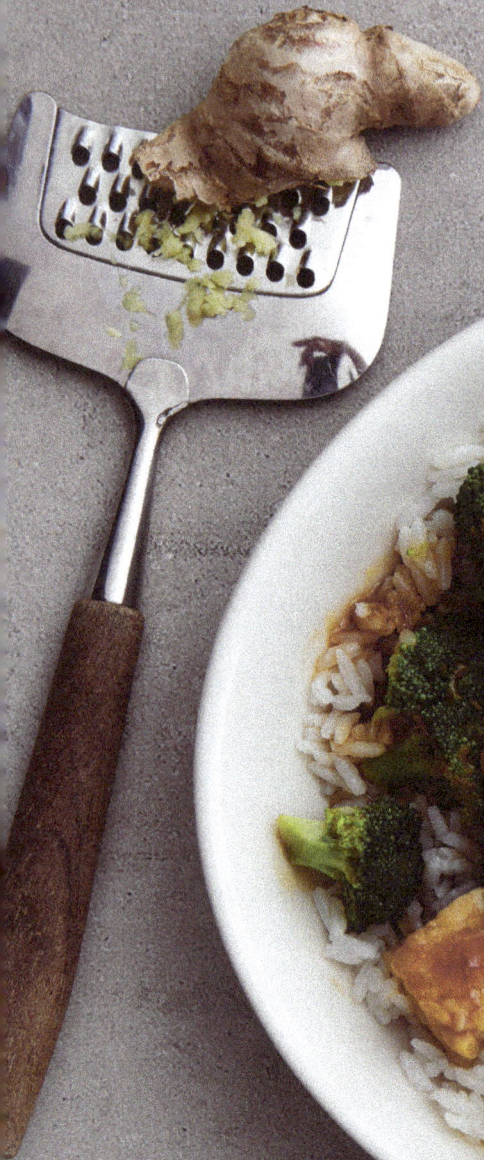

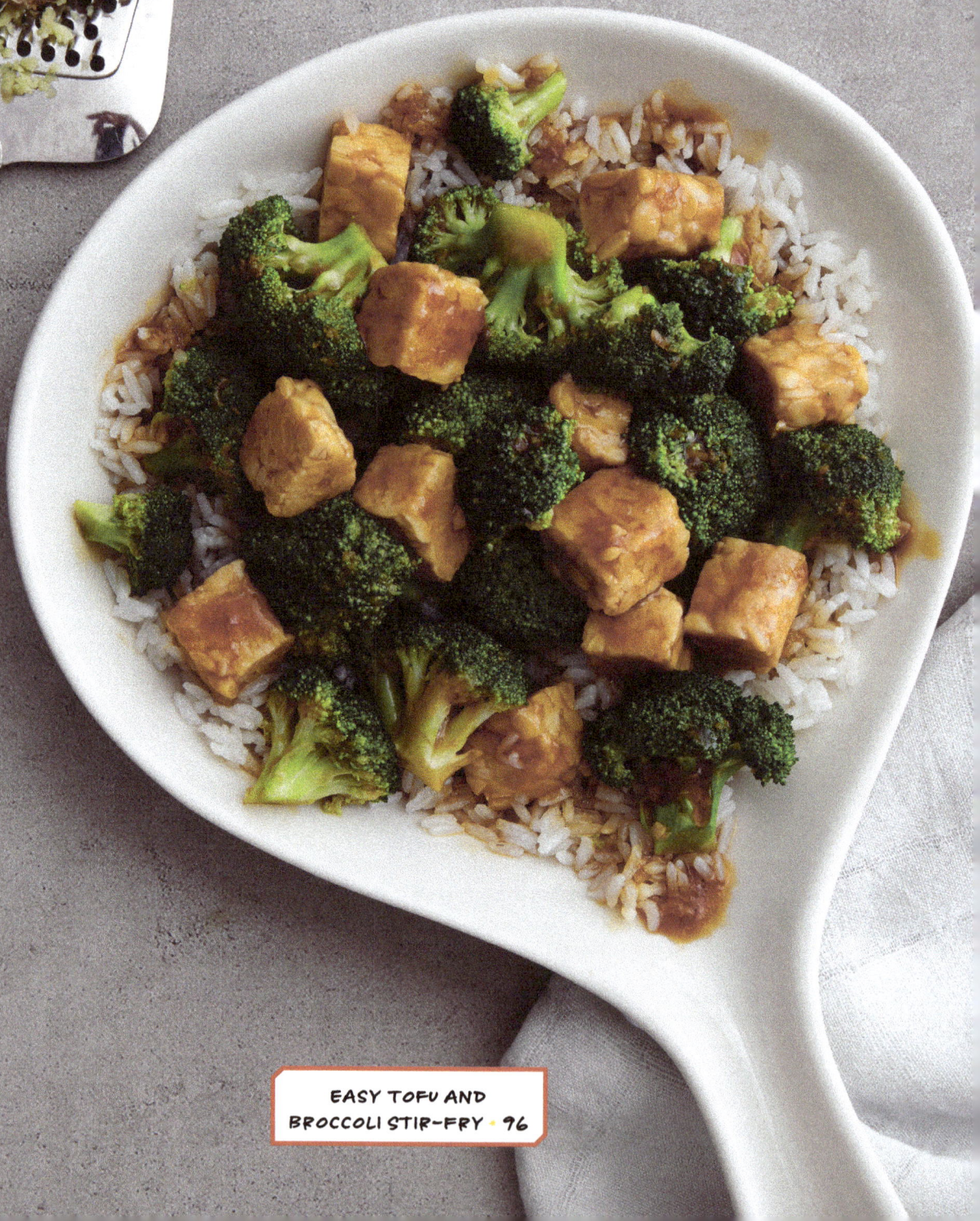

Chapter Six

VEGETARIAN MAINS AND SIDE DISHES

96 **Easy Tofu and Broccoli Stir-Fry**

97 **Parmesan Baked Asparagus and Eggs**

98 **Lentil Sloppy Joes**

99 **Swiss Mushroom Quiche**

100 **The Best Black Bean Burgers**

102 **Easy Grandma Pie Pizza**

103 **Pierogi with Fried Onions and Cabbage**

104 **Baked BBQ Tofu and Broccoli**

105 **Pinto Bean and Spinach Quesadillas**

106 **Buffalo Cauliflower Tacos**

107 **Lasagna-Stuffed Zucchini Boats**

108 **Baked Sweet Potatoes with Cinnamon Honey**

109 **Garlic Roasted Potatoes with Rosemary**

110 **Cheesy Roasted Cauliflower**

111 **Crispy Baked Carrot Fries**

112 **Summer Squash Marinara**

113 **Summer Squash "Pasta" with Peas**

114 **Parmesan Baked Artichoke Hearts**

115 **Wilted Balsamic Spinach**

116 **Garlicky Peas and Mushrooms**

117 **Chili Butter Corn on the Cob**

Easy Tofu and Broccoli Stir-Fry

PREP TIME *10 MINUTES*   **COOK TIME** *25 MINUTES*   **SERVES** *4*

DAIRY-FREE   QUICK PREP   VEGETARIAN

You won't want to order takeout again after you see how easy this stir-fry recipe is to prepare. The tofu is tender and soaks up the flavor of the sauce, which is sweet and tangy. It will be sure to please the whole family, even the kiddos.

Main Ingredients

1 pound extra-firm tofu, drained and cut into ¾-inch cubes

¼ cup reduced-sodium soy sauce

4 garlic cloves, minced

1 tablespoon minced ginger

3 cups broccoli florets

Pantry Staples

7 tablespoons vegetable oil, divided

Salt and black pepper

1. In a large skillet over medium heat, heat 3 tablespoons of olive oil. Add the tofu to the pan and season lightly with salt and pepper. Cook, turning occasionally, until browned on all sides, 10 to 15 minutes.

2. While the tofu is cooking, in a small bowl, combine the soy sauce, garlic, ginger, remaining 4 tablespoons of vegetable oil, and pepper to taste. Reserve 2 tablespoons of the sauce and set aside in a small bowl.

3. When the tofu is browned, transfer it to a plate and set aside. Add the broccoli and soy sauce mixture to the skillet and toss to ensure all the broccoli is evenly coated. Raise the heat to medium-high and cook until the sauce begins to reduce, 4 to 5 minutes. Cover the pan and cook until the broccoli is tender, 3 to 5 minutes. Return the tofu to the pan, add the reserved 2 tablespoons of sauce, and stir until the tofu is coated with sauce. Divide the mixture evenly between 4 bowls.

Ingredient Tip: If your family wants to spice up this recipe, add chili flakes or sriracha sauce before serving.

Serving Suggestion: This recipe is delicious served over steamed brown or white rice, or another grain of your choice.

Parmesan Baked Asparagus and Eggs

PREP TIME *10 MINUTES* **COOK TIME** *18 MINUTES* **SERVES** *4*

30 MINUTES OR LESS   **GLUTEN-FREE**   **ONE PAN**   **QUICK PREP**   **VEGETARIAN**

Asparagus with eggs is a low-carb meal packed with bold flavor. The asparagus is flavored with lemon juice and garlic powder, then topped with eggs over easy. Add toast to the side for something to dip into those delicious runny egg yolks!

Main Ingredients

1½ pounds asparagus, trimmed

Juice of 1 lemon

1 teaspoon garlic powder

⅓ cup shredded vegetarian Parmesan cheese

4 large eggs

Pantry Staples

1 tablespoon olive oil

Salt and black pepper

1. Preheat the oven to 400°F. Line a sheet pan with parchment paper or spray it with cooking spray.

2. Toss the asparagus with the lemon juice and olive oil. Arrange the asparagus on the prepared sheet pan and season with the garlic powder, salt, and black pepper.

3. Bake for 10 minutes. Sprinkle with the Parmesan cheese. Crack the eggs over the asparagus and bake for another 8 minutes, or until the eggs are set and cooked to your liking. Season with more salt and black pepper, transfer to plates, and serve.

Ingredient Tip: When buying asparagus, look for stalks that are bright green with a purplish tinge. They should have firm stems that are not limp or woody.

Lentil Sloppy Joes

PREP TIME 5 MINUTES   **COOK TIME 30 MINUTES**   **SERVES 4**

DAIRY-FREE   ONE POT   QUICK PREP   VEGAN

Sloppy Joes can easily be made into a vegan version using lentils. This lentil-based sloppy joe recipe will have your family convinced they are eating meat!

Main Ingredients

1 cup lentils, rinsed

1 medium onion, chopped

1 (8-ounce) can tomato sauce

⅓ cup barbecue sauce

4 hamburger buns

Pantry Staples

1 tablespoon olive oil

Salt and black pepper

1. In a medium saucepan over medium-high heat, bring the lentils and 2 cups of water to a boil. Lower the heat to low and cook until the lentils are tender, about 10 minutes. Drain any excess liquid, transfer to a bowl, and set aside.

2. In the same saucepan over medium-high heat, heat the olive oil. Add the onion and sauté, stirring frequently, until it starts to brown, 6 to 8 minutes.

3. Add the tomato sauce, barbecue sauce, and lentils and stir well. Bring to a simmer, lower the heat to low, cover, and cook until heated through, about 10 minutes. Add more water to reach the desired consistency, if necessary. Season with salt and black pepper.

4. Spoon the lentil mixture onto the buns and serve.

Serving Suggestion: For an easy weeknight dinner, serve these sandwiches with pickles and coleslaw. If your family is into spicy food, serve hot sauce on the side.

Swiss Mushroom Quiche

PREP TIME *10 MINUTES*   **COOK TIME** *45 MINUTES*   **SERVES** *6*

QUICK PREP   VEGETARIAN

Quiche is such a versatile meal. It's a great choice for breakfast, lunch, or dinner, and you can add many different ingredients and flavoring agents. For this recipe, the quiche is flavored with mushrooms and cheese. A refrigerated piecrust is used for simple meal preparation.

Main Ingredients

8 ounces white mushrooms, sliced

4 eggs

1½ cups milk

1 (9- to 10-inch) refrigerated piecrust

1 cup shredded Swiss cheese

Pantry Staples

1 tablespoon olive oil

Salt and black pepper

1. Preheat the oven to 375°F.

2. In a large nonstick skillet over medium heat, heat the olive oil. Add the mushrooms and sauté until soft, about 10 minutes.

3. In a medium bowl, beat together the eggs and milk. Season with salt and black pepper. Add the mushrooms and mix until combined.

4. Line a 9-inch pie plate with the refrigerated piecrust. Sprinkle the cheese on the bottom of the crust and pour the egg mixture over the cheese. Bake for 35 minutes, or until the top is golden and puffy.

5. Let cool, cut into slices, and serve.

Cooking Tip: Refrigerated piecrust is an easy way to get a quiche in the oven quickly. Make sure to bring the crust to room temperature before using. Use the tines of a fork to pinch the edge of the crust to the pie plate. If the edge of the crust browns too quickly, tent it with thin strips of aluminum foil.

The Best Black Bean Burgers

PREP TIME *15 MINUTES*   **COOK TIME** *20 MINUTES*

CHILL TIME *30 MINUTES*   **SERVES** *6*

DAIRY-FREE   **ONE PAN**   **VEGAN**

These black bean burgers are an absolutely delicious vegetable burger option! The avocado acts as a binder so you don't have to use eggs, and it also makes a great burger topping. The burgers are flavored with chili powder, avocado, and salt and pepper.

Main Ingredients

2 (15-ounce) cans black beans, drained and rinsed

¾ cup seasoned bread crumbs

2 ripe avocados, pitted and peeled, half mashed and half sliced, divided

1 to 2 tablespoons chili powder

6 hamburger buns

Pantry Staples

2 to 3 tablespoons olive oil

Salt and black pepper

1. In a medium bowl, lightly mash the beans with a fork. Add the bread crumbs and mashed avocados and stir until combined. Add the chili powder, using less or more depending on how spicy you like your burgers, and stir until combined. If the mixture seems too dry, add 1 tablespoon of water to the mixture.

2. Using wet hands, shape the black bean mixture into 6 patties. Place the patties on a plate, cover with plastic wrap, and refrigerate for 30 minutes.

3. Heat 2 tablespoons of olive oil in a large nonstick skillet over medium-high heat. Cook half the patties until they are lightly browned and crispy, about 5 minutes on each side. Transfer the bean burgers to a plate, cover with aluminum foil, and keep warm. Repeat with the remaining patties and add the remaining 1 tablespoon of olive oil to the pan if necessary.

4. Place the black bean burgers on the buns and top with avocado slices. Season with salt and black pepper to taste and serve immediately.

Leftover Tip: You can make the burgers in advance and freeze them. Cook the patties, let them cool completely, then place them on a sheet pan and freeze them in a single layer for 2 to 3 hours. At that point they can be stored in an airtight container or wrapped in plastic wrap and frozen for up to 1 month. To reheat, cook the burgers in the microwave oven on high for about 90 seconds or in a nonstick pan coated with oil over medium heat for about 5 minutes on each side.

Serving Suggestion: Don't forget your burger toppings! Pile on the lettuce, tomatoes, ketchup, and pickles.

Easy Grandma Pie Pizza

PREP TIME *20 MINUTES*   **COOK TIME** *15 MINUTES*   **SERVES** *6*
PLUS 1 HOUR RESTING TIME

ONE PAN   VEGETARIAN

There is nothing better than pizza right out of the oven. Grandma pie pizza is unusual in that it is typically a rectangle, and the cheese is placed on the bottom and the sauce is on top, which keeps the crust nice and crispy. This is a great family dinner to make, because everyone can help roll out the dough.

Main Ingredients

1 pound refrigerated pizza dough

1 (14-ounce) can crushed tomatoes

1 teaspoon garlic powder

12 ounces shredded mozzarella cheese

¼ cup chopped fresh basil

Pantry Ingredients

½ teaspoon salt

¼ teaspoon black pepper

2 tablespoons olive oil, divided

1. Let the dough sit out at room temperature, still wrapped in plastic, for 1 hour, until it rises a bit and gets more pliable.

2. In a medium bowl, mix together the crushed tomatoes, garlic powder, salt, and black pepper and set aside.

3. Preheat the oven to 500°F. Position an oven rack at the lowest level. Brush a large sheet pan with 1 tablespoon of olive oil.

4. Roll out the pizza dough to fit it into the sheet pan. Lightly brush the dough with the remaining 1 tablespoon of olive oil.

5. Sprinkle the dough with the cheese. Spoon the sauce over the cheese and sprinkle with the basil.

6. Bake for 15 minutes, or until the crust turns golden brown and the sauce and cheese are bubbling. Let cool for 10 minutes, cut into squares, and serve.

Ingredient Tip: If you do not have fresh basil, use 2 tablespoons of dried basil instead. The flavor will still be wonderful.

Pierogi with Fried Onions and Cabbage

PREP TIME *10 MINUTES* **COOK TIME** *20 MINUTES* **SERVES** *4*

30 MINUTES OR LESS   **ONE PAN**   **QUICK PREP**   **VEGETARIAN**

Grocery stores typically carry several brands of delicious frozen pierogi in a variety of flavors. The addition of some sautéed onions and cabbage turns the dumplings into a comforting and complete meal without the hassle of anything made from scratch. Plain potato or cheese pierogi go nicely with the vegetables and are a sure bet for even the pickiest palate.

Main Ingredients

1 medium onion, finely chopped

½ head cabbage, shredded, or 1 (8-ounce) packaged shredded cabbage

1 (16-ounce) package frozen pierogi

½ cup sour cream

2 tablespoons chopped fresh parsley

Pantry Staples

2 tablespoons olive oil

Salt and black pepper

1. In a large nonstick skillet over medium heat, heat the olive oil. Add the onion and cook, stirring occasionally, until translucent, about 5 minutes. Add the cabbage, mix well, and cook until the cabbage is tender and cooked through, about 10 minutes.

2. Add the pierogi to the skillet, lower the heat to low, and cook, stirring occasionally, until the pierogi are fully cooked, about 6 minutes.

3. Add salt and black pepper to taste, garnish with sour cream and fresh parsley, and serve.

Ingredient Tip: To save time, use a bag of preshredded cabbage, which can be found at most grocery stores in the produce section.

Baked BBQ Tofu and Broccoli

PREP TIME *30 MINUTES*   **COOK TIME** *40 MINUTES*   **SERVES** *4*

DAIRY-FREE   GLUTEN-FREE   ONE PAN   VEGAN

Dinners baked on a sheet pan are always nice because they are easy to clean up, and this crispy baked BBQ tofu with broccoli is no exception! Tofu has a very mild flavor and will taste like the marinade or seasoning you cook it in. The tofu prepared in this recipe offers the bold, smoky flavor of the barbecue sauce. This meal is the perfect solution to your next "Meatless Monday" meal!

Main Ingredients

1 (14-ounce) block extra-firm tofu, drained, patted dry, pressed, and cut into bite-size pieces

1 tablespoon barbecue seasoning

1 tablespoon cornstarch

2 cups broccoli florets

¼ cup barbecue sauce

Pantry Staples

2 tablespoons olive oil, divided

Salt and black pepper

1. Preheat the oven to 400°F. Line a large sheet pan with parchment paper or spray it with cooking spray.

2. In a medium bowl, mix together the tofu cubes, barbecue seasoning, and cornstarch and 1 tablespoon of olive oil until evenly coated.

3. Place the tofu in a single layer on one side of the sheet pan. Bake for 20 minutes. Remove the pan from the oven and turn over the tofu.

4. In a medium bowl, toss the broccoli florets with the remaining 1 tablespoon of olive oil and season with salt and black pepper to taste. Arrange the broccoli on the other half of the sheet pan.

5. Return the pan to the oven and bake for another 20 minutes, or until the tofu is crispy and the broccoli is tender.

6. Toss the tofu with the barbecue sauce and serve with the broccoli.

Ingredient Tip: Buy extra-firm tofu, which has the least amount of moisture, and you will achieve a nice crispy crust after baking.

Pinto Bean and Spinach Quesadillas

PREP TIME 5 MINUTES   **COOK TIME 25 MINUTES**   **SERVES 4**

30 MINUTES OR LESS   ONE PAN   QUICK PREP   VEGETARIAN

These hearty quesadillas are stuffed with beans and spinach, which makes them super healthy. They are so hearty you won't even need a side dish and can serve them as a stand-alone meal, though you might want to serve them with some salsa or sour cream on the side for an extra treat.

Main Ingredients

1 (15-ounce) can pinto beans, drained and rinsed

5 ounces fresh baby spinach

1 tablespoon chili powder

8 large burrito-size tortillas

8 ounces shredded cheddar cheese

Pantry Staples

2 tablespoons olive oil

Salt and black pepper

Nonstick cooking spray

1. In a large nonstick skillet over medium heat, heat the olive oil. Add the beans, spinach, and chili powder and cook until the spinach is softened but not mushy, about 5 minutes. Season with salt and black pepper to taste. Transfer to a bowl and set aside.

2. Wipe out the skillet with a paper towel and coat it with cooking spray. Set the pan over medium heat. Place 1 tortilla in the skillet and spoon ¼ of the bean and spinach mixture on top. Sprinkle with ¼ of the cheese and top with another tortilla. Cook until golden brown on the bottom, about 2 minutes. Turn over the quesadilla and cook on the other side until golden brown, about 2 minutes. Transfer the quesadilla to a plate and keep warm in the oven set to the lowest temperature.

3. Repeat to make three more quesadillas.

4. Cut the quesadillas into wedges and serve.

Substitution Tip: Black beans or white cannellini beans can be used in place of pinto beans.

Buffalo Cauliflower Tacos

PREP TIME *10 MINUTES*   **COOK TIME** *15 MINUTES*   **SERVES** *6*

30 MINUTES OR LESS   **ONE PAN**   **QUICK PREP**   **VEGETARIAN**

If you are looking for a flavorful vegetarian taco option, this cauliflower is the perfect solution. The cauliflower is flavored with a tangy Buffalo sauce and topped with avocado and ranch dressing. But you can really get creative and add any toppings you like such as cheddar cheese, chopped cilantro, shredded lettuce, and chopped tomatoes.

Main Ingredients

1 small head cauliflower, cut into bite-size pieces

1/3 cup Buffalo sauce

12 (6-inch) flour tortillas, warmed

2 avocados, pitted, peeled, and chopped

1/2 cup ranch dressing

Pantry Staples

2 tablespoons olive oil

1 teaspoon salt

1/2 teaspoon black pepper

1. Preheat the oven to 450°F. Line a sheet pan with parchment paper or spray it with cooking spray.

2. Toss the cauliflower and olive oil on the prepared sheet pan. Sprinkle with the salt and black pepper and toss until combined. Spread out the cauliflower in a single layer on the sheet pan.

3. Roast for 15 minutes, or until the cauliflower is tender and starts to brown. Remove the cauliflower from oven and toss with the Buffalo sauce right on the sheet pan. Return the pan to the oven and bake for 5 minutes more, or until the cauliflower is crispy.

4. To assemble the tacos, spoon the Buffalo cauliflower equally onto the tortillas and top with the chopped avocados. Drizzle with the ranch dressing and serve.

Serving Suggestion: For a real feast, serve these tacos with some Crispy Baked Carrot Fries (page 111) or Chili Butter Corn on the Cob (page 117).

Lasagna-Stuffed Zucchini Boats

PREP TIME 20 MINUTES   **COOK TIME 20 MINUTES**   **SERVES 4**

GLUTEN-FREE   ONE PAN   VEGETARIAN

Change up how you serve lasagna to your family with these Lasagna-Stuffed Zucchini Boats. Your family won't find any lasagna noodles in this meal! But they will still enjoy the delicious flavors of traditional lasagna, just served in a refreshing zucchini half.

Main Ingredients

4 medium zucchini, halved lengthwise

1 cup marinara sauce, divided

1 cup part-skim ricotta cheese

1 large egg, beaten

1 cup shredded Italian cheese blend

Pantry Staples

½ teaspoon salt

Nonstick cooking spray

1 tablespoon olive oil

1. Preheat the oven to 400°F. Scoop out the center flesh and seeds of the zucchini, leaving some around the edges to keep the boat sturdy. Sprinkle the zucchini with the salt, flip them over onto a plate, and set aside for about 10 minutes so they release their liquid.

2. Pat the zucchini dry and place them in a baking dish or on a sheet pan that has been sprayed with cooking spray. In a small saucepan over medium heat, cook the marinara sauce until it is simmering.

3. In a small bowl, mix together the ricotta cheese and egg. Spoon some of the ricotta mixture into each zucchini boat and top with the marinara sauce. Sprinkle with the shredded cheese.

4. Bake for 15 to 20 minutes, or until the zucchini is tender and the cheese is melted and golden brown. Serve hot.

Serving Suggestion: For a heartier vegetarian dinner, served this zucchini dish with some Tomato-Basil Gnocchi (page 48) or Black Pepper Spaghetti with Garlic and Parmesan (page 50).

Cooking Tip: While you can make these in the oven as described, in the middle of summer you can also make these on the grill in a disposable cooking pan. Keep an eye on the cooking time, as the heat from gas grills can vary compared to an oven.

Baked Sweet Potatoes with Cinnamon Honey

PREP TIME *10 MINUTES*   **COOK TIME** *50 MINUTES*   **SERVES** *4*

GLUTEN-FREE   ONE PAN   QUICK PREP   VEGETARIAN

This baked sweet potato recipe is a simplified version of the traditional sweet potato casserole most commonly served at holiday meals. This recipe offers a healthier solution that requires very little preparation.

Main Ingredients

4 medium sweet potatoes, scrubbed and patted dry

2 tablespoons salted butter, softened

1½ tablespoons honey

½ teaspoon ground cinnamon

Pantry Staples

Salt and black pepper

1. Preheat the oven to 400°F.

2. Wrap each sweet potato individually in aluminum foil and, using a fork, prick holes in each potato. Place on a sheet pan.

3. Bake for 45 to 50 minutes, or until the sweet potatoes are fork-tender.

4. While the potatoes are baking, in a small bowl mix together the butter, honey, and cinnamon.

5. Set the baked sweet potatoes on a plate and let cool for 5 to 10 minutes. Remove the foil and split open each potato diagonally. Divide the butter mixture equally between the potatoes and season with salt and black pepper to taste. Serve immediately.

Leftover Tip: If you have any leftover baked sweet potatoes you can mash them or add them to a hash and serve it with breakfast.

Garlic Roasted Potatoes with Rosemary

PREP TIME *10 MINUTES*   **COOK TIME** *30 MINUTES*   **SERVES** *4 TO 6*

DAIRY-FREE   GLUTEN-FREE   ONE PAN   QUICK PREP   VEGAN

Roasted potatoes are a staple in most households—they go with most types of meat, poultry, and seafood. For extra nutrition (and to simplify prep), you can skip peeling the potatoes. You can just roast them with the skins left on. The herbs and seasonings can be modified to your liking—consider a substitution such as dill, paprika, or chili powder. You can make this with russet or Yukon Gold potatoes.

Main Ingredients

2 pounds red-skinned potatoes, scrubbed and cut into 1- to 2-inch cubes

1 tablespoon dried rosemary

1 teaspoon garlic powder

Pantry Staples

Nonstick cooking spray

2 tablespoons olive oil

½ teaspoon salt

½ teaspoon black pepper

1. Preheat the oven to 425°F. Spray a large sheet pan with cooking spray.

2. In a large bowl, toss the potatoes, rosemary, garlic powder, olive oil, salt, and black pepper until evenly coated.

3. Spread out the seasoned potatoes on the prepared sheet pan. Bake for 20 minutes.

4. Flip the potatoes and continue to bake for 10 more minutes, or until the potatoes are crispy and golden brown. Let cool slightly and serve.

Cooking Tip: Make sure to spread the potatoes out in a single layer on the sheet pan. This will help make them nice and crispy. If you cannot fit them on one pan, divide them between two sheet pans and bake as instructed.

Cheesy Roasted Cauliflower

PREP TIME *10 MINUTES* **COOK TIME** *35 MINUTES* **SERVES** *4*

GLUTEN-FREE ONE PAN QUICK PREP VEGETARIAN

Roasting cauliflower offers a delicious flavor, because it brings out its amazing sweetness. It's also a neutral-flavored vegetable that takes on flavors from other ingredients, so in this case the garlic, lemon juice, and olive oil give it a light, fresh taste. The melted cheese amps it up a notch.

Main Ingredients

1 medium head of cauliflower, trimmed and cut into florets

2 garlic cloves, minced

Juice of 1 lemon

1 cup shredded cheddar cheese

Pantry Staples

2 tablespoons olive oil

Salt and black pepper

1. Preheat the oven to 400°F. Line a large sheet pan with parchment paper or spray it with cooking spray.

2. In a large bowl, mix together the cauliflower, garlic, lemon juice, and olive oil. Sprinkle with salt and black pepper and stir until combined.

3. Spread out the cauliflower in a single layer on the prepared sheet pan.

4. Roast for 30 minutes, or until the cauliflower turns golden brown, stirring once in the middle of cooking.

5. Remove from the oven and sprinkle with the cheddar cheese. Return to the oven and roast for 5 minutes, or until the cheese is melted and bubbly. Serve hot.

Substitution Tip: Use mozzarella, Parmesan, or Gruyère cheese. Any of these will give the dish a new flavor.

Crispy Baked Carrot Fries

PREP TIME *10 MINUTES*   COOK TIME *20 MINUTES*   SERVES *4*

**30 MINUTES OR LESS   DAIRY-FREE   GLUTEN-FREE   ONE PAN
QUICK PREP   VEGAN**

If you have selective eaters, here's a great way to get them to eat carrots. They are so good, no one will realize that the carrot fries are healthy. And go ahead and serve these with ketchup, ranch dressing, or your favorite dipping sauce to make them even more mouthwatering.

Main Ingredients

1½ pounds carrots, peeled and cut into thin 3-inch sticks

1 tablespoon cornstarch

1 teaspoon garlic powder

1 to 2 tablespoons dried parsley

Pantry Staples

1½ tablespoons olive oil

1 teaspoon salt

½ teaspoon black pepper

1. Preheat the oven to 425°F. Line a large sheet pan with parchment paper or spray it with cooking spray.

2. In a large bowl, mix together the carrots, cornstarch, garlic powder, olive oil, salt, and black pepper.

3. Spread out the carrots in a single layer on the prepared sheet pan. Bake for 20 minutes, or until the carrots are crispy and browned.

4. Sprinkle with 1 to 2 tablespoons of dried parsley, as desired, and serve hot.

Substitution Tip: If you'd like a more flavor-filled version of this recipe, sprinkle the carrots with cayenne pepper instead of black pepper and substitute chopped fresh cilantro for the parsley.

Summer Squash Marinara

PREP TIME *10 MINUTES*   **COOK TIME** *20 MINUTES*   **SERVES** *4 TO 6*

30 MINUTES OR LESS   **GLUTEN-FREE**   **ONE PAN**   **QUICK PREP**   **VEGETARIAN**

This easy summer side dish offers zucchini seasoned with garlic and tomatoes and topped with Italian seasoning and Parmesan cheese. It pairs well with a variety of mains like poultry, beef, or seafood.

Main Ingredients

3 medium zucchini, cut into ½-inch slices

3 garlic cloves, minced

1 (14-ounce) can crushed tomatoes

1 tablespoon Italian seasoning

½ cup grated vegetarian Parmesan cheese

Pantry Staples

2 tablespoons olive oil

1. In a large nonstick skillet over medium-high heat, heat the olive oil. Arrange the zucchini slices in the pan in a single layer, add the garlic, and let cook undisturbed until they start to brown, 3 to 5 minutes. Turn the slices over and cook until brown. (If all the zucchini does not fit in your pan, you can cook it in two batches.)

2. Lower the heat to low and pour the crushed tomatoes and Italian seasoning over the zucchini. Stir gently, cover the pan, and simmer until the zucchini is cooked to your desired doneness, 10 to 15 minutes.

3. Top with the grated Parmesan and serve hot.

Leftover Tip: Try heating this up the next day and mixing it with penne pasta for a great leftover lunch or dinner.

Summer Squash "Pasta" with Peas

PREP TIME *10 MINUTES* **COOK TIME** *10 MINUTES* **SERVES** *4*

30 MINUTES OR LESS **ONE PAN** **QUICK PREP** **VEGETARIAN**

This vegetable-based dish offers a fresh flavor that will make your family forget they're eating vegetables and not real noodles. The spiralized squash is a great base for a sauce and can serve as a side dish or as a simple meal all on its own.

Main Ingredients

1 garlic clove, minced

3 medium summer squash or zucchini, spiralized

1 cup cooked peas, frozen or fresh

1 to 2 tablespoons freshly squeezed lemon juice

⅓ cup shaved vegetarian Parmesan cheese, plus more for garnish

Pantry Staples

¼ cup olive oil

Salt and black pepper

1. In a large skillet over medium heat, heat the olive oil. Add the garlic and cook until lightly browned, 2 to 4 minutes.

2. Add the squash and cook, stirring frequently, until tender, 2 to 4 minutes.

3. Add the peas, 1 tablespoon of lemon juice, salt and pepper to taste, and Parmesan cheese and stir until combined. Taste and add more lemon juice if desired.

4. Divide the squash noodles evenly between 4 bowls. Garnish with additional shaved Parmesan and black pepper.

Cooking Tip: For a quick solution to cooking the peas, prepare them in the microwave. Place the peas in a microwave-safe bowl and cover with water. Microwave on high until they are tender, 2 to 3 minutes.

Ingredient Tip: If you don't have a spiralizer, use a vegetable peeler to peel the zucchini into long ribbons. Stack the ribbons on top of each other and, using a chef's knife, cut them into thin strips to make "noodles." If the ribbons are too slippery, stack about half and cut them in batches.

Parmesan Baked Artichoke Hearts

PREP TIME 10 MINUTES   **COOK TIME** 20 MINUTES   **SERVES** 4

30 MINUTES OR LESS   ONE PAN   QUICK PREP   VEGETARIAN

Creating stuffed artichoke recipes can be a lot of work, though the flavors are wonderful. This recipe uses artichoke hearts, which are much easier to cook and just as delicious!

Main Ingredients

2 (14-ounce) cans artichoke hearts

1 large lemon

½ cup Italian-seasoned bread crumbs

½ cup shredded vegetarian Parmesan cheese

3 tablespoons chopped fresh parsley

Pantry Staples

Nonstick cooking spray

2 tablespoons olive oil

½ teaspoon black pepper

1. Preheat the oven to 400°F. Spray a baking dish with cooking spray.

2. Arrange the artichokes, cut-side up, in a single layer in the baking dish. Squeeze the lemon juice over the top.

3. In a medium skillet over medium-high heat, heat the olive oil. Add the bread crumbs and toast them, stirring constantly, until golden brown, 3 to 4 minutes. Remove the pan from the heat.

4. Stir in the Parmesan cheese, black pepper, and parsley and carefully pour the mixture over the artichoke hearts. Bake for 10 to 15 minutes, or until the top is golden brown. Serve hot.

Serving Suggestion: These artichokes make a great side dish with the Turkey Cutlets with White Wine and Mushrooms (page 72).

Wilted Balsamic Spinach

PREP TIME *5 MINUTES*   **COOK TIME** *10 MINUTES*   **SERVES** *4*

30 MINUTES OR LESS   **DAIRY-FREE**   **GLUTEN-FREE**   **ONE PAN**
QUICK PREP   **VEGAN**

Sautéed spinach is a quick, easy to cook, and deliciously healthy vegetable dish for your family meal. The balsamic vinegar and garlic give the spinach just the right amount of flavor without being overpowering. You can double the batch to produce leftovers to use in omelets or serve with meals for upcoming days.

Main Ingredients

2 garlic cloves, minced

10 ounces fresh baby spinach

2 tablespoons balsamic vinegar

Pantry Staples

2 tablespoons olive oil

Salt and black pepper

1. In a large nonstick skillet over medium heat, heat the olive oil. Add the garlic and cook until it turns golden, about 2 minutes.

2. Add the spinach and balsamic vinegar and toss well until combined. Cook, stirring occasionally, until the greens start to wilt, 3 to 5 minutes. Season with salt and black pepper and serve immediately.

Serving Suggestion: Make this side dish to accompany the Lemon and Herb Scallops recipe (page 93), though it's versatile enough to serve with any poultry, meat, or seafood dish.

Garlicky Peas and Mushrooms

PREP TIME 10 MINUTES   **COOK TIME** 15 MINUTES   **SERVES** 6

**30 MINUTES OR LESS   DAIRY-FREE   GLUTEN-FREE   ONE PAN
QUICK PREP   VEGAN**

This recipe is great any time of year for family dinners or holiday gatherings. It's an excellent solution to get your family to eat peas! The secret ingredient that makes this taste so good is just a little white wine. You can use broth or water instead, but wine really gives the vegetables that extra layer of flavor.

Main Ingredients

3 garlic cloves, minced

8 to 10 ounces white button mushrooms, sliced

1 (16-ounce) package frozen peas

½ cup white wine

Pantry Staples

2 tablespoons olive oil

Salt and black pepper

1. In a large nonstick skillet over medium-high heat, heat the olive oil. Add the garlic and mushrooms and cook, stirring occasionally, until the mushrooms soften and the juices are released, about 5 minutes.

2. Stir in the peas and white wine and cook, stirring frequently, until the peas and mushrooms are tender, about 10 minutes. Season with salt and black pepper to taste and serve immediately.

Leftover Tip: Heat up any leftovers with some butter and white rice. It makes a tasty vegetarian lunch for the next day.

Chili Butter Corn on the Cob

PREP TIME *10 MINUTES*   **COOK TIME** *15 MINUTES*   **SERVES** *4*

30 MINUTES OR LESS   GLUTEN-FREE   ONE POT   QUICK PREP   VEGETARIAN

Corn is a super easy side dish to make and is featured on many families' tables or at group gatherings throughout the summer months. This extremely simple corn recipe offers bold spices, dominated by the chili powder.

Main Ingredients

4 ears of corn, shucked

2 tablespoons butter, melted

1 tablespoon chili powder

Pantry Staples

Salt and black pepper

1. Fill a large pot halfway with salted water and bring to a boil over medium-high heat.

2. Place the corn in the pot and cook until tender, about 8 minutes. Transfer the corn to a serving platter.

3. Drizzle the butter over the corn and sprinkle with the chili powder. Season with extra salt and black pepper to taste. Serve hot.

Cooking Tip: The easiest way to shuck corn is to pull the husks all the way down to reveal the cob. Remove all the silk tassels and rip off the husks. Remove any stray silk strands still sticking to the kernels. Make sure to have a garbage bag ready to get rid of the husks and silk strands. If this is too much work, make sure to buy the corn already shucked.

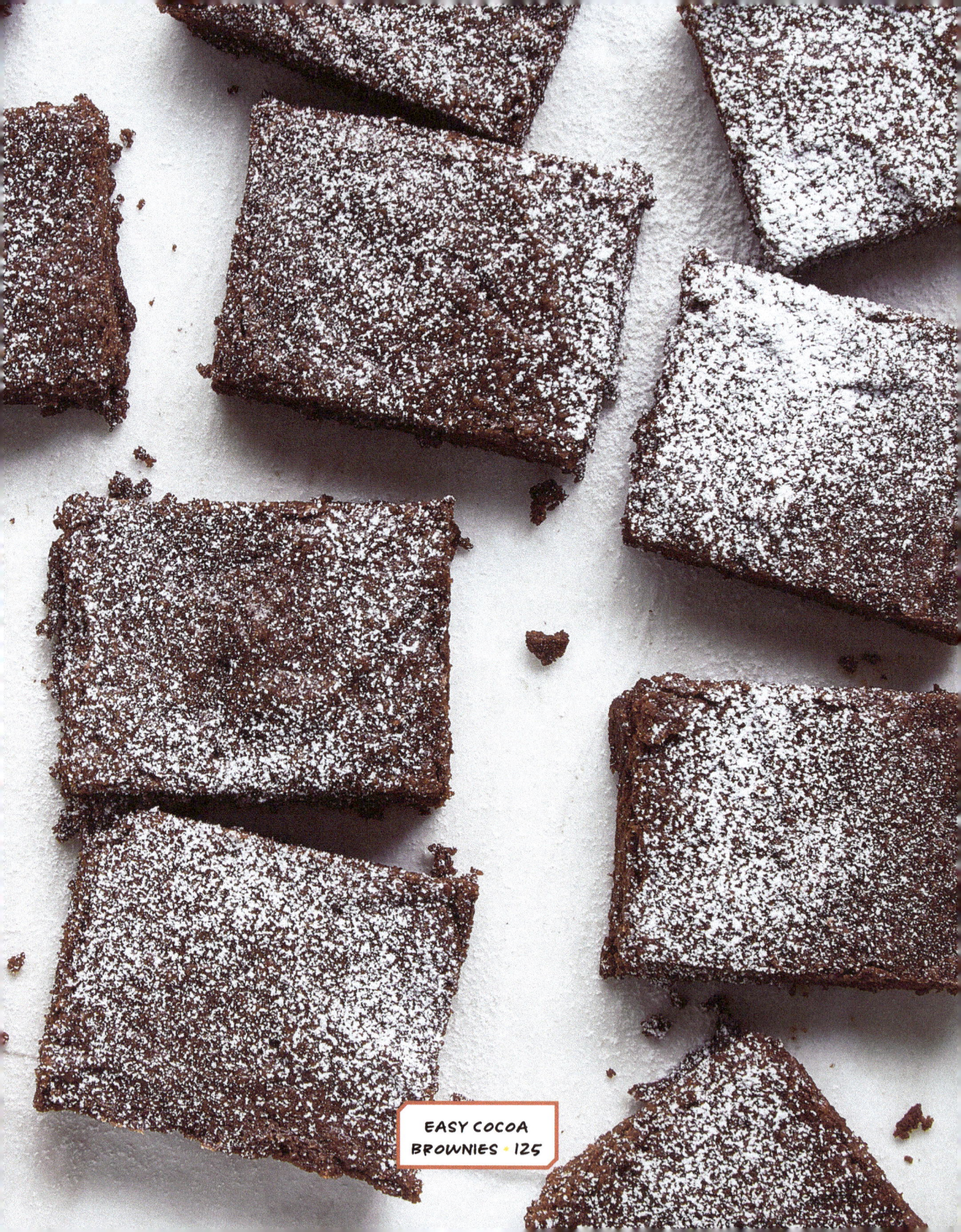

EASY COCOA
BROWNIES • 125

Chapter Seven

DESSERTS

120 **Honey-Lime Fruit Salad**

121 **Old-Fashioned Ambrosia**

122 **Chocolate-Dipped Strawberries**

123 **Pear Bread Pudding**

124 **Raspberry-Filled Butter Cookies**

125 **Easy Cocoa Brownies**

126 **Luscious Lemon Pie**

127 **Brown Sugar Apple Galette**

128 **Peach and Granola Crisp**

Honey-Lime Fruit Salad

PREP TIME *10 MINUTES*   **SERVES** *4 TO 6*

30 MINUTES OR LESS   DAIRY-FREE   GLUTEN-FREE   QUICK PREP   VEGETARIAN

Light and refreshing, this dessert salad is a nice way to end a meal. It's great for a barbecue or party alfresco. Wherever you serve it, you won't find any leftovers! Make a double recipe to enjoy with breakfast the next day.

Main Ingredients

2 cups strawberries, halved

½ cantaloupe, cut into 1-inch chunks

2 cups grapes

Juice of 1 large lime

2 tablespoons honey

1. In a medium bowl, mix the strawberries, cantaloupe, and grapes.

2. In a small bowl, whisk together the lime juice and honey. Drizzle the mixture over the fruit and toss lightly. Serve at room temperature or chilled.

Substitution Tip: Follow the season and make this fruit salad with whatever you can find at your farmers' market. Strawberries can be replaced with blueberries, blackberries, or raspberries. Cantaloupe can be exchanged for another melon or 2 cups of diced peaches or orange sections.

Old-Fashioned Ambrosia

PREP TIME *10 MINUTES*　　　**CHILL TIME** *1 HOUR*　　　**SERVES** *6*

30 MINUTES OR LESS　　GLUTEN-FREE　　QUICK PREP

Perhaps this is a recipe you remember enjoying as a child, but you haven't seen it in ages. It's time to give it another try, as you will be surprised just how delicious this creamy fruit salad is! If you have never had it before, be sure to try it.

Main Ingredients

1 (15-ounce) can mandarin orange segments, drained

1 (15 ounce) can crushed pineapple, drained

1 cup mini marshmallows

1 cup sour cream

1 (10-ounce) jar maraschino cherries, drained and stems removed

In a medium bowl, mix together the mandarin oranges, pineapple, marshmallows, and sour cream. Add the cherries and stir until combined. Cover the bowl with plastic wrap and refrigerate for 1 hour before serving.

Ingredient Tip: Canned fruit is packed in either fruit juice or a sugar syrup. It's up to you to choose the variety that most suits your taste. Fruit packed in sugar syrup will be much sweeter.

Chocolate-Dipped Strawberries

PREP TIME *30 MINUTES*   **SERVES** *6*

GLUTEN-FREE   VEGETARIAN

Chocolate-dipped strawberries are always a crowd-pleaser. Plus, this recipe brings in an extra fruit serving at dessert time. Bonus for sure! This recipe steps up the standard chocolate-dipped recipe a notch by adding crushed pistachios.

Main Ingredients

1 pound strawberries

8 ounces semisweet chocolate chips, plus extra if needed

1 teaspoon canola oil

½ cup crushed pistachios

1. Line a large sheet pan with wax paper or parchment paper.

2. Wash and dry the strawberries and let them sit out at room temperature for 30 minutes to make sure any excess moisture evaporates.

3. In a microwave-safe bowl, combine the chocolate chips and canola oil. Microwave in 20-second intervals, stirring after each interval, until melted, smooth, and shiny, 60 to 80 seconds total.

4. Holding a strawberry by the stem, dip it into the chocolate, letting any excess chocolate drip into the bowl. Dip the tip of the strawberry into the nuts and place the strawberry on the sheet pan. Repeat with the remaining strawberries. Refrigerate the dipped strawberries for about 30 minutes or let them sit at room temperature for 1 hour, or until the chocolate is set.

5. Serve at room temperature.

Substitution Tip: The pistachios can be swapped out for another type of crushed nuts, such as walnuts or almonds. For another topping variation, you could use colored sprinkles or shredded coconut.

Pear Bread Pudding

PREP TIME *15 MINUTES* **COOK TIME** *50 MINUTES* **SERVES** *6*

ONE PAN **QUICK PREP** **VEGETARIAN**

Autumn typically launches the pear and apple recipes. This bread pudding recipe is a delicious way to use any extra pears you might have picked up. Anjou, Bosc, or Bartlett pears are all good in this recipe.

Main Ingredients

2 cups whole milk

½ cup sugar, plus 2 tablespoons

3 large eggs, beaten

8 slices white bread, cut into bite-size cubes

2 large pears, peeled, cored, and chopped

Pantry Staples

Nonstick cooking spray

1. Preheat the oven to 350°F. Spray an 8- to 10-inch square sheet pan with cooking spray.

2. In a medium bowl, whisk together the milk, ½ cup of sugar, and eggs.

3. Toss together the bread cubes and pears on the sheet pan. Pour the milk and egg mixture over the top, making sure all the bread cubes are covered, and let sit for 5 minutes.

4. Bake for 30 minutes. Sprinkle the remaining 2 tablespoons of sugar over the top and continue to bake for 20 more minutes, or until a toothpick inserted in the middle comes out clean and the top is golden brown. Spoon into bowls and serve.

Serving Suggestion: To dress this dessert up, serve it warm with ice cream and/or whipped cream.

Substitution Tip: Feel free to substitute apples, too, for the pears because apple bread pudding is just as tasty.

Raspberry-Filled Butter Cookies

PREP TIME 30 MINUTES   **COOK TIME 15 MINUTES**   **SERVES 4 TO 6**

ONE PAN   **VEGETARIAN**

It is possible to make cookies from scratch with only 5 ingredients! These raspberry-filled cookies will remind you of something you picked up from your local bakery. Sprinkle a little powdered sugar on top to make them a bit fancier. They will look like they came from the bakery but taste even better.

Main Ingredients

½ cup butter, softened

1 teaspoon vanilla extract

⅓ cup sugar

1 cup all-purpose flour

3 tablespoons raspberry jam

1. In a medium bowl, using an electric hand mixer or a wooden spoon, beat together the butter, vanilla extract, and sugar until well incorporated. Gradually add the flour and mix until the dough is crumbly.

2. Form the dough into a ball, wrap it in plastic wrap, and refrigerate for at least 1 hour or up to overnight.

3. Preheat the oven to 350°F. Line a sheet pan with parchment paper or spray it with cooking spray.

4. Using your hands, roll the dough into 12 to 16 (1-inch) balls and place them on the prepared sheet pan, spacing them about 2 inches apart. Using your thumb or a wooden spoon, make a little well in the middle of each ball. Fill each well equally with the jam, making sure not to overfill.

5. Bake for 13 to 16 minutes, or until the cookies turn golden around the edges. Let cool for 20 to 30 minutes and serve.

Substitution Tip: You can replace the raspberry jam with any other flavor you like. You can try apricot, grape, or strawberry jam to change these cookies up a bit.

Easy Cocoa Brownies

PREP TIME *10 MINUTES*   **COOK TIME** *25 MINUTES*   **SERVES** *12*

ONE PAN   QUICK PREP   VEGETARIAN

Why make brownies from a boxed mix when you can make these home-made ones in the same amount of time? They are incredibly simple and offer a delicious chocolate flavor. To make a big batch, just double the recipe and use a bigger sheet pan. They will take about 10 minutes longer to bake. Put the extras in lunch boxes or share them with friends.

Main Ingredients

1 cup all-purpose flour

1 cup sugar

½ cup unsweetened cocoa powder

2 eggs

Powdered sugar, for dusting

Pantry Staples

½ teaspoon salt

½ cup olive oil

1. Preheat the oven to 350°F. Line an 8-inch square baking dish with parchment paper (see Cooking Tip) or spray it with cooking spray.

2. In a medium bowl, whisk together the flour, sugar, cocoa powder, and salt.

3. In a small bowl, whisk together the eggs and olive oil. Add the wet mixture to the dry mixture and stir until combined, making sure to scrape down the sides of the bowl. Spread the batter evenly into the pan.

4. Bake for 25 minutes, or until the brownies are set in the center. Lift the brownies out of the pan using the edges of the parchment paper as handles. Place on a cutting board to cool for about 20 minutes. Dust with powdered sugar, then cut into squares and serve.

Cooking Tip: To line the pan with parchment paper, cut a square that is larger than the baking pan. You'll use the edges as handles to remove the brownies. Press creases in the parchment paper at the edges to make it fit into the bottom of the pan. You can also spray the pan with cooking spray before lining with parchment, which will help keep the parchment paper in place.

Ingredient Tip: If you really want to spoil your family, stir 1 cup of chocolate chips into the batter before baking.

Luscious Lemon Pie

PREP TIME *10 MINUTES*   **COOK TIME** *25 MINUTES*   **SERVES** *6*

ONE PAN   QUICK PREP   VEGETARIAN

This pie omits the meringue topping included in traditional lemon pies. The recipe uses sweetened whipped cream instead. It doesn't take long to make this pie, but there is some cooling time, so you will need to keep that in mind.

Main Ingredients

1 (9-inch) refrigerated piecrust

1 (14-ounce) can sweetened condensed milk

3 egg yolks

½ cup freshly squeezed lemon juice

Sweetened whipped cream, for topping

1. Preheat the oven to 450°F.

2. Line a 9-inch pie pan with the piecrust. Gently prick the piecrust all over with a fork. Bake for about 10 minutes, or until the crust is lightly golden. Let cool completely, about 30 minutes.

3. Lower oven temperature to 350°F.

4. In a medium bowl, whisk together the condensed milk, egg yolks, and lemon juice. Pour the filling into the baked crust.

5. Bake for 12 to 14 minutes, or until the filling is set. Let the pie cool in the refrigerator until it is no longer warm, about 2 hours. Cover the top of the pie with whipped cream. Cut into slices and serve.

Cooking Tip: Homemade whipped cream is incredibly easy to prepare, so you might consider giving it a shot. Simply beat some whipping cream with an electric mixer. Add a few spoonfuls of sugar (depending on how sweet you like it) before beating the cream. To make things super easy, you can use canned whipped cream to top off this pie, but make sure not to top it until right before serving.

Brown Sugar Apple Galette

PREP TIME *10 MINUTES* **COOK TIME** *30 MINUTES* **SERVES** *6*

30 MINUTES OR LESS **ONE PAN** **QUICK PREP** **VEGETARIAN**

There is nothing better than the smell of an apple dessert cooking in in the fall. An added bonus is one that cooks quickly, and this one bakes in 30 minutes for nearly instant gratification. Keep things simple by using refrigerated piecrust.

Main Ingredients

3 medium apples, peeled, cored, and thinly sliced

½ cup packed brown sugar

1 refrigerated piecrust

1 egg yolk, beaten

2 tablespoons granulated sugar

1. Preheat the oven to 400°F. Line a baking pan with parchment paper or spray it with cooking spray.

2. In a medium bowl, mix together the apples and brown sugar.

3. Unroll the piecrust onto the prepared baking pan. Pile the apples in the center of the piecrust and turn the edges over the apples. Brush the crust with the egg yolk and sprinkle the galette with the sugar.

4. Bake for 25 to 30 minutes, or until the apples are tender and the crust is golden. Let cool for 20 minutes. Cut into slices and serve.

Ingredient Tip: Aim to use Granny Smith apples for this recipe because they are tart and keep their shape. Jonagold, Cortland, and Honeycrisp apples are also great choices for the same reason. If you would like less work in this recipe, you can keep the skins on and have a more rustic galette.

Serving Suggestion: Serve this galette with a scoop of ice cream on top for your next dinner party, or just because.

Peach and Granola Crisp

PREP TIME *15 MINUTES*   **COOK TIME** *50 MINUTES*   **SERVES** *6*

ONE PAN   QUICK PREP   VEGETARIAN

If your family prefers a fresh fruit dessert over chocolate, this recipe is for you! No crust or breading for this recipe—it's a simple crisp with peaches and a buttery sugar and granola topping. Easy to get on the table, it can turn any night into a special occasion.

Main Ingredients

6 peaches, pitted and sliced

¼ cup sugar

2 cups granola

2 tablespoons salted butter, melted

3 tablespoons slivered almonds

1. Preheat the oven to 350°F.

2. In an 8-inch baking dish, toss together the peaches and sugar. Bake for 40 minutes, or until the peaches are bubbling and most of the liquid has evaporated.

3. In a medium bowl, toss together the granola, melted butter, and almonds.

4. Sprinkle the granola over the peaches and bake for another 10 minutes or until the granola is golden brown. Cool for 10 minutes and serve.

Serving Suggestion: Top the warm crisp with vanilla ice cream.

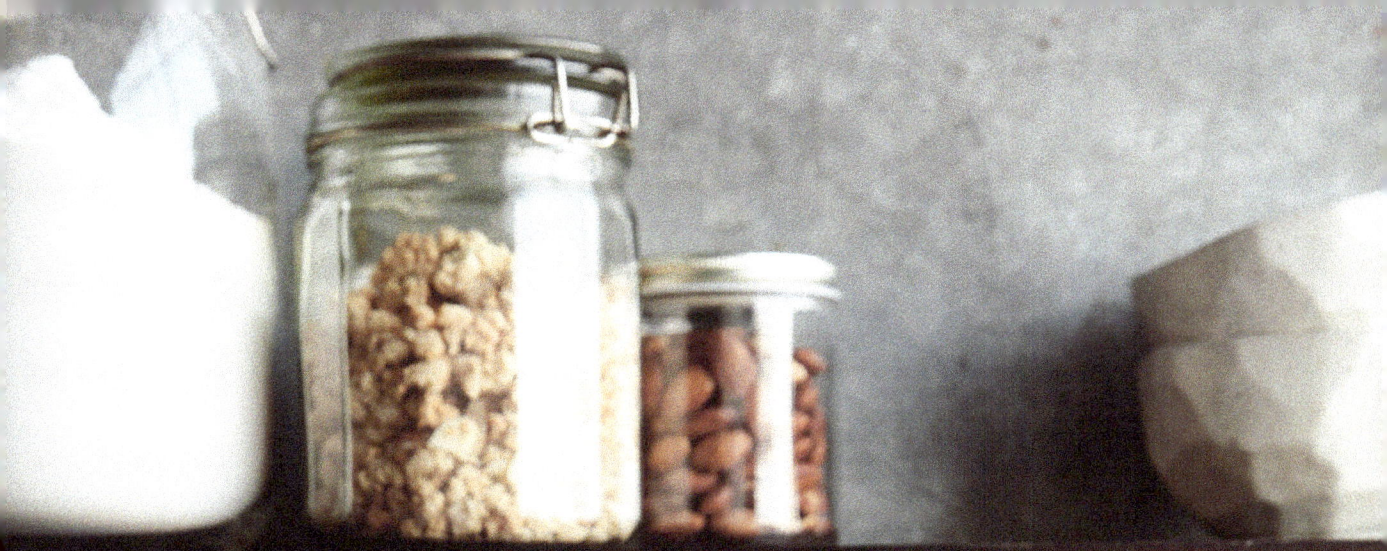

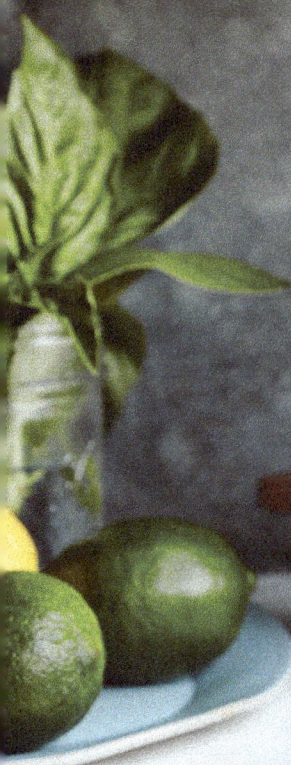

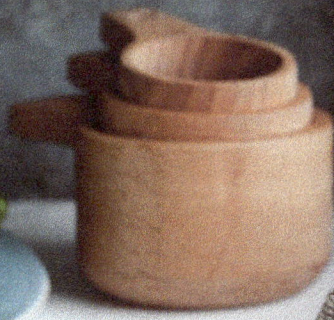

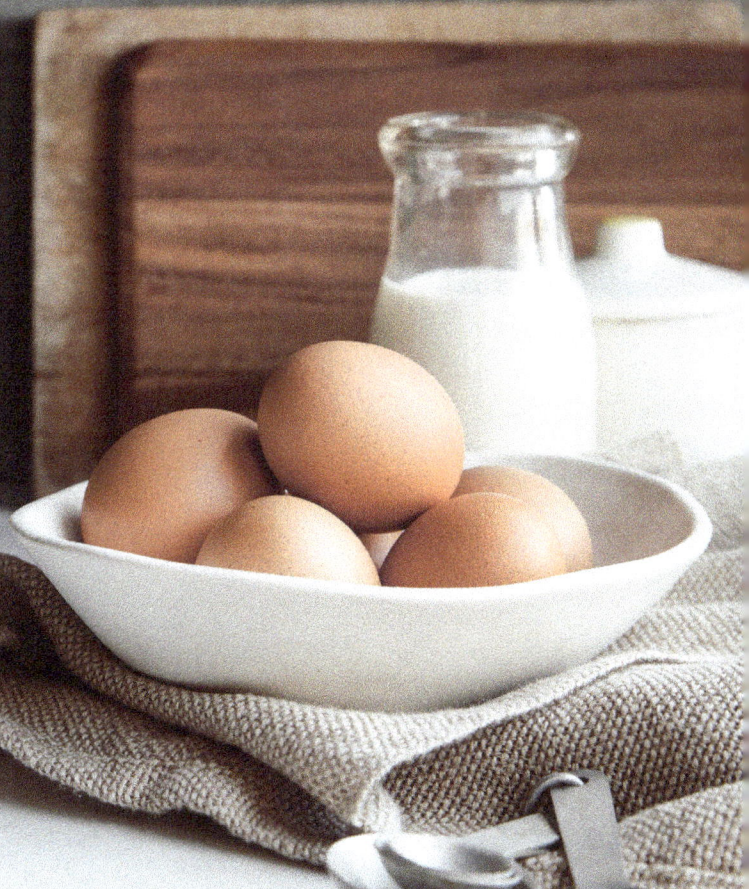

Measurement Conversions

Volume Equivalents	U.S. STANDARD	U.S. STANDARD (OUNCES)	METRIC (APPROXIMATE)
Liquid	2 tablespoons	1 fl. oz.	30 mL
	¼ cup	2 fl. oz.	60 mL
	½ cup	4 fl. oz.	120 mL
	1 cup	8 fl. oz.	240 mL
	1½ cups	12 fl. oz.	355 mL
	2 cups or 1 pint	16 fl. oz.	475 mL
	4 cups or 1 quart	32 fl. oz.	1 L
	1 gallon	128 fl. oz.	4 L
Dry	⅛ teaspoon	—	0.5 mL
	¼ teaspoon	—	1 mL
	½ teaspoon	—	2 mL
	¾ teaspoon	—	4 mL
	1 teaspoon	—	5 mL
	1 tablespoon	—	15 mL
	¼ cup	—	59 mL
	⅓ cup	—	79 mL
	½ cup	—	118 mL
	⅔ cup	—	156 mL
	¾ cup	—	177 mL
	1 cup	—	235 mL
	2 cups or 1 pint	—	475 mL
	3 cups	—	700 mL
	4 cups or 1 quart	—	1 L
	½ gallon	—	2 L
	1 gallon	—	4 L

Oven Temperatures

FAHRENHEIT	CELSIUS (APPROXIMATE)
250°F	120°C
300°F	150°C
325°F	165°C
350°F	180°C
375°F	190°C
400°F	200°C
425°F	220°C
450°F	230°C

Weight Equivalents

U.S. STANDARD	METRIC (APPROXIMATE)
½ ounce	15 g
1 ounce	30 g
2 ounces	60 g
4 ounces	115 g
8 ounces	225 g
12 ounces	340 g
16 ounces or 1 pound	455 g

Index

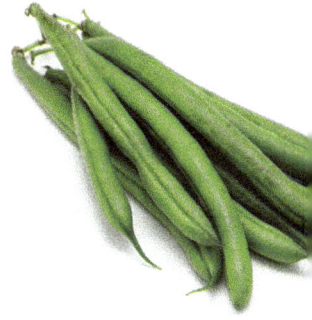

A

Ambrosia, Old-Fashioned, 121
Apple Galette, Brown Sugar, 127
Artichoke Hearts, Parmesan Baked, 114
Arugula
  Arugula Shrimp Salad with Lemon Olive Oil, 41
  Chicken Milanese with Arugula, 68
  Summer Arugula Salad with Watermelon, 35
Asparagus and Eggs, Parmesan Baked, 97
Avocados
  Chocolate-Avocado Smoothie, 22
  Easy Tuna and Avocado Panzanella Salad, 42
  Hearty Salmon Avocado Toast, 18
  Shrimp and Avocado Tostadas, 92

B

Bacon
  Blue Cheese and Bacon Wedge Salad, 44
  Penne Florentine with Bacon, 55
  Sheet Pan Breakfast Bake, 17
  Spinach Salad with Eggs and Bacon, 43
Balsamic Spinach, Wilted, 115
Bananas
  Baked Oat Banana Muffins, 19
  Yogurt Banana Split, 21
Barley Bowls, California Veggie, 59
Basil
  Caprese Corn and Tomato Salad, 37
  Tomato-Basil Gnocchi, 48

Beans
  The Best Black Bean Burgers, 100–101
  Chicken and White Bean Chili, 33
  Ham, Bean, and Potato Soup, 30
  Pinto Bean and Spinach Quesadillas, 105
  Quinoa with Spicy Black Beans and
    Sausage, 63
  Simple Baked Black Bean Huevos Rancheros, 14
  Simple Beef and Black Bean Chili, 34
  30-Minute Minestrone, 27
Beef
  Chili-Rubbed Steak and Red Pepper
    Kebabs, 78
  Easy Baked Ziti Casserole, 54
  French Onion Burgers, 75
  Ground Beef and String Bean Stir-Fry, 74
  Pan-Seared Sirloin Tips with Mushrooms, 76
  Peppery Chicken-Fried Cube Steaks, 79
  Red Gravy Pot Roast, 81
  Simple Beef and Black Bean Chili, 34
  Soy-Marinated Flank Steak, 77
  The Ultimate Philly Cheesesteak, 80
Beets and Goat Cheese, Baby
    Greens Salad with, 40
Bell peppers
  Chili-Rubbed Steak and Red Pepper
    Kebabs, 78
  Hawaiian Pork and Pineapple Kebabs, 83
  Pork Chop Fajita Skillet, 85

Berries
Chocolate-Dipped Strawberries, 122
Raspberry-Filled Butter Cookies, 124
Strawberry Cheesecake Toast, 20
Strawberry, Spinach, and Mozzarella
Salad, 36
Black Pepper Spaghetti with Garlic
and Parmesan, 50
Bread Pudding, Pear, 123
Breakfasts
Baked Egg and Sausage Breakfast Taquitos, 15
Baked Oat Banana Muffins, 19
Chocolate-Avocado Smoothie, 22
Hearty Salmon Avocado Toast, 18
Savory Breakfast Egg Muffins, 16
Sheet Pan Breakfast Bake, 17
Simple Baked Black Bean Huevos
Rancheros, 14
Simple Buttermilk Pancakes, 23
Strawberry Cheesecake Toast, 20
Yogurt Banana Split, 21
Broccoli
Baked BBQ Tofu and Broccoli, 104
Easy Tofu and Broccoli Stir-Fry, 96
Penne with Broccoli Pesto, 52
Brownies, Easy Cocoa, 125
Brown Sugar Apple Galette, 127
Buffalo Cauliflower Tacos, 106
Burgers
The Best Black Bean Burgers, 100–101
French Onion Burgers, 75
Buttermilk Pancakes, Simple, 23
Butternut squash
Easiest Butternut Squash Risotto, 58
Sweet and Savory Butternut Squash Soup, 26

C

Cabbage, Pierogi with Fried Onions, 103
Caprese Corn and Tomato Salad, 37
Carrot Fries, Crispy Baked, 111
Cauliflower
Buffalo Cauliflower Tacos, 106
Cheesy Roasted Cauliflower, 110

Cheese
Baby Greens Salad with Beets
and Goat Cheese, 40
Baked Chicken Thighs with
Tomatoes and Feta, 69
Baked Egg and Sausage Breakfast
Taquitos, 15
Black Pepper Spaghetti with
Garlic and Parmesan, 50
Blue Cheese and Bacon Wedge Salad, 44
Caprese Corn and Tomato Salad, 37
Cheesy Roasted Cauliflower, 110
Easiest Baked Mac and Cheese, 51
Easy Baked Ziti Casserole, 54
Lasagna-Stuffed Zucchini Boats, 107
Parmesan Baked Artichoke Hearts, 114
Parmesan Baked Asparagus and Eggs, 97
Pinto Bean and Spinach Quesadillas, 105
Roasted Veggie Salad with Feta, 39
Savory Breakfast Egg Muffins, 16
Simple Baked Black Bean Huevos
Rancheros, 14
Strawberry, Spinach, and Mozzarella Salad, 36
Swiss Mushroom Quiche, 99
The Ultimate Philly Cheesesteak, 80
Chicken
Baked Chicken Thighs with
Tomatoes and Feta, 69
Chicken and White Bean Chili, 33
Chicken Enchiladas Verde, 67
Chicken Milanese with Arugula, 68
Couscous with Lemon Chicken and Olives, 62
Lemon Chicken Orzo Soup, 28
Lemon Oregano Chicken Skewers
with Yogurt Sauce, 66
Savory Chicken, Tomato, and
Mushroom Stew, 31
Sunday Roast Chicken Dinner, 70
Super Easy Chicken Fried Rice, 57
Chili. See Soups, stews, and chilis
Chili Butter Corn on the Cob, 117
Chili-Rubbed Steak and Red Pepper
Kebabs, 78

Chocolate
  Chocolate-Avocado Smoothie, 22
  Chocolate-Dipped Strawberries, 122
  Easy Cocoa Brownies, 125
Cinnamon Honey, Baked Sweet Potatoes with, 108
Cookies, Raspberry-Filled Butter, 124
Corn
  Caprese Corn and Tomato Salad, 37
  Chili Butter Corn on the Cob, 117
Couscous with Lemon Chicken and Olives, 62

D

Dairy-free
  Arugula Shrimp Salad with Lemon Olive Oil, 41
  Baked BBQ Tofu and Broccoli, 104
  Baked Oat Banana Muffins, 19
  The Best Black Bean Burgers, 100–101
  Chicken and White Bean Chili, 33
  Chicken Milanese with Arugula, 68
  Chili-Rubbed Steak and Red Pepper Kebabs, 78
  Couscous with Lemon Chicken and Olives, 62
  Crispy Baked Carrot Fries, 111
  Easy Tofu and Broccoli Stir-Fry, 96
  Easy Tuna and Avocado Panzanella Salad, 42
  Garlicky Peas and Mushrooms, 116
  Garlic Roasted Potatoes with Rosemary, 109
  Ground Beef and String Bean Stir-Fry, 74
  Ham, Bean, and Potato Soup, 30
  Hawaiian Pork and Pineapple Kebabs, 83
  Hearty Salmon Avocado Toast, 18
  Honey-Lime Fruit Salad, 120
  Lemon Chicken Orzo Soup, 28
  Lemon-Dill Salmon Packet, 89
  Lemon Pepper Pork Tenderloin with
    Roasted Root Vegetables, 86–87
  Lentil Sloppy Joes, 98
  Open-Faced Pulled Pork Sandwiches, 84
  Pan-Seared Sirloin Tips with Mushrooms, 76
  Penne Florentine with Bacon, 55
  Pork Chop Fajita Skillet, 85
  Quinoa with Spicy Black Beans and Sausage, 63
  Red Gravy Pot Roast, 81
  Rigatoni with Sausage and Chunky
    Tomato Sauce, 56

Roasted BBQ Turkey Drumsticks, 71
  Savory Chicken, Tomato, and
    Mushroom Stew, 31
  Seared Tuna Steaks with Slaw, 91
  Sheet Pan Baked Fish and Chips, 90
  Sheet Pan Lemon-Garlic Salmon
    and Veggie Bowl, 88
  Sheet Pan Sausage, Poblano
    Pepper, and Potatoes, 82
  Shrimp Orzo Skillet, 53
  Simple Beef and Black Bean Chili, 34
  Smoked Sausage and Potato Stew, 32
  Soy-Marinated Flank Steak, 77
  Spicy Peanut Noodles, 49
  Sunday Roast Chicken Dinner, 70
  Super Easy Chicken Fried Rice, 57
  Turkey Cutlets with White Wine
    and Mushrooms, 72–73
  Wilted Balsamic Spinach, 115
Desserts
  Brown Sugar Apple Galette, 127
  Chocolate-Dipped Strawberries, 122
  Easy Cocoa Brownies, 125
  Honey-Lime Fruit Salad, 120
  Luscious Lemon Pie, 126
  Old-Fashioned Ambrosia, 121
  Peach and Granola Crisp, 128
  Pear Bread Pudding, 123
  Raspberry-Filled Butter Cookies, 124
Dill Salmon Packet, Lemon, 89

E

Eggs
  Baked Egg and Sausage Breakfast
    Taquitos, 15
  Parmesan Baked Asparagus
    and Eggs, 97
  Savory Breakfast Egg Muffins, 16
  Sheet Pan Breakfast Bake, 17
  Simple Baked Black Bean Huevos
    Rancheros, 14
  Spinach Salad with Eggs and Bacon, 43
Enchiladas Verde, Chicken, 67
Equipment, 10–11

F

Farro with Zucchini and Walnuts, 60–61
Fish and seafood
  Arugula Shrimp Salad with Lemon Olive Oil, 41
  Easy Tuna and Avocado Panzanella Salad, 42
  Hearty Salmon Avocado Toast, 18
  Lemon and Herb Scallops, 93
  Lemon-Dill Salmon Packet, 89
  Seared Tuna Steaks with Slaw, 91
  Sheet Pan Baked Fish and Chips, 90
  Sheet Pan Lemon-Garlic Salmon
    and Veggie Bowl, 88
  Shrimp and Avocado Tostadas, 92
  Shrimp Orzo Skillet, 53
Fries, Crispy Baked Carrot, 111
Fruit Salad, Honey Lime, 120

G

Garlic
  Black Pepper Spaghetti with
    Garlic and Parmesan, 50
  Garlicky Peas and Mushrooms, 116
  Garlic Roasted Potatoes with Rosemary, 109
  Sheet Pan Lemon-Garlic Salmon
    and Veggie Bowl, 88
Gluten-free
  Arugula Shrimp Salad with Lemon Olive Oil, 41
  Baby Greens Salad with Beets
    and Goat Cheese, 40
  Baked BBQ Tofu and Broccoli, 104
  Baked Chicken Thighs with
    Tomatoes and Feta, 69
  Baked Egg and Sausage Breakfast Taquitos, 15
  Baked Sweet Potatoes with
    Cinnamon Honey, 108
  Blue Cheese and Bacon Wedge Salad, 44
  Caprese Corn and Tomato Salad, 37
  Cheesy Roasted Cauliflower, 110
  Chicken and White Bean Chili, 33
  Chicken Enchiladas Verde, 67
  Chili Butter Corn on the Cob, 117
  Chili-Rubbed Steak and Red Pepper Kebabs, 78

Chocolate-Avocado Smoothie, 22
Chocolate-Dipped Strawberries, 122
Chopped Mediterranean Salad, 38
Crispy Baked Carrot Fries, 111
Easiest Butternut Squash Risotto, 58
Garlicky Peas and Mushrooms, 116
Garlic Roasted Potatoes with Rosemary, 109
Ham, Bean, and Potato Soup, 30
Hawaiian Pork and Pineapple Kebabs, 83
Honey-Lime Fruit Salad, 120
Lasagna-Stuffed Zucchini Boats, 107
Lemon and Herb Scallops, 93
Lemon-Dill Salmon Packet, 89
Lemon Oregano Chicken Skewers
  with Yogurt Sauce, 66
Lemon Pepper Pork Tenderloin with
  Roasted Root Vegetables, 86–87
Old-Fashioned Ambrosia, 121
Pan-Seared Sirloin Tips with Mushrooms, 76
Parmesan Baked Asparagus and Eggs, 97
Pork Chop Fajita Skillet, 85
Quinoa with Spicy Black Beans and
  Sausage, 63
Red Gravy Pot Roast, 81
Roasted BBQ Turkey Drumsticks, 71
Savory Chicken, Tomato, and
  Mushroom Stew, 31
Sheet Pan Breakfast Bake, 17
Sheet Pan Sausage, Poblano
  Pepper, and Potatoes, 82
Shrimp and Avocado Tostadas, 92
Simple Baked Black Bean Huevos Rancheros, 14
Simple Beef and Black Bean Chili, 34
Smoked Sausage and Potato Stew, 32
Spinach Salad with Eggs and Bacon, 43
Strawberry, Spinach, and Mozzarella Salad, 36
Summer Arugula Salad with Watermelon, 35
Summer Squash Marinara, 112
Sunday Roast Chicken Dinner, 70
Super Easy Chicken Fried Rice, 57
Sweet and Savory Butternut Squash Soup, 26
Wilted Balsamic Spinach, 115
Yogurt Banana Split, 21

Granola Crisp, Peach and, 128
Greens Salad with Beets and Goat
        Cheese, Baby, 40

H

Ham
    Ham, Bean, and Potato Soup, 30
    Savory Breakfast Egg Muffins, 16
Honey
    Baked Sweet Potatoes with
        Cinnamon Honey, 108
    Honey-Lime Fruit Salad, 120

K

Kale, Tortellini Soup with Italian
        Sausage and Baby, 29
Kebabs and skewers
    Chili-Rubbed Steak and Red Pepper Kebabs, 78
    Hawaiian Pork and Pineapple Kebabs, 83
    Lemon Oregano Chicken Skewers
        with Yogurt Sauce, 66

L

Lasagna-Stuffed Zucchini Boats, 107
Lemons
    Arugula Shrimp Salad with Lemon Olive Oil, 41
    Couscous with Lemon Chicken and Olives, 62
    Lemon and Herb Scallops, 93
    Lemon Chicken Orzo Soup, 28
    Lemon-Dill Salmon Packet, 89
    Lemon Oregano Chicken Skewers
        with Yogurt Sauce, 66
    Luscious Lemon Pie, 126
    Sheet Pan Lemon-Garlic Salmon
        and Veggie Bowl, 88
Lentil Sloppy Joes, 98
Lime Fruit Salad, Honey, 120

M

Meal planning, 6–9
Muffins
    Baked Oat Banana Muffins, 19
    Savory Breakfast Egg Muffins, 16

Mushrooms
    Garlicky Peas and Mushrooms, 116
    Pan-Seared Sirloin Tips with Mushrooms, 76
    Savory Chicken, Tomato, and
        Mushroom Stew, 31
    Swiss Mushroom Quiche, 99
    Turkey Cutlets with White Wine
        and Mushrooms, 72–73

O

Oat Banana Muffins, Baked, 19
Olive Oil, Arugula Shrimp Salad with Lemon, 41
Olives, Couscous with Lemon Chicken and, 62
One pot/pan
    Arugula Shrimp Salad with Lemon Olive Oil, 41
    Baked BBQ Tofu and Broccoli, 104
    Baked Sweet Potatoes with
        Cinnamon Honey, 108
    The Best Black Bean Burgers, 100–101
    Black Pepper Spaghetti with
        Garlic and Parmesan, 50
    Brown Sugar Apple Galette, 127
    Buffalo Cauliflower Tacos, 106
    Caprese Corn and Tomato Salad, 37
    Cheesy Roasted Cauliflower, 110
    Chicken and White Bean Chili, 33
    Chicken Enchiladas Verde, 67
    Chicken Milanese with Arugula, 68
    Chili Butter Corn on the Cob, 117
    Chili-Rubbed Steak and Red Pepper Kebabs, 78
    Chocolate-Avocado Smoothie, 22
    Couscous with Lemon Chicken and Olives, 62
    Crispy Baked Carrot Fries, 111
    Easiest Butternut Squash Risotto, 58
    Easy Cocoa Brownies, 125
    Easy Grandma Pie Pizza, 102
    French Onion Burgers, 75
    Garlicky Peas and Mushrooms, 116
    Garlic Roasted Potatoes with Rosemary, 109
    Ground Beef and String Bean Stir-Fry, 74
    Ham, Bean, and Potato Soup, 30
    Hawaiian Pork and Pineapple Kebabs, 83
    Hearty Salmon Avocado Toast, 18

One pot/pan (*continued*)
  Lasagna-Stuffed Zucchini Boats, 107
  Lemon and Herb Scallops, 93
  Lemon Chicken Orzo Soup, 28
  Lemon-Dill Salmon Packet, 89
  Lemon Oregano Chicken Skewers
      with Yogurt Sauce, 66
  Lentil Sloppy Joes, 98
  Luscious Lemon Pie, 126
  Open-Faced Pulled Pork Sandwiches, 84
  Pan-Seared Sirloin Tips with Mushrooms, 76
  Parmesan Baked Artichoke Hearts, 114
  Parmesan Baked Asparagus and Eggs, 97
  Peach and Granola Crisp, 128
  Pear Bread Pudding, 123
  Penne Florentine with Bacon, 55
  Peppery Chicken-Fried Cube Steaks, 79
  Pierogi with Fried Onions and Cabbage, 103
  Pinto Bean and Spinach Quesadillas, 105
  Pork Chop Fajita Skillet, 85
  Raspberry-Filled Butter Cookies, 124
  Red Gravy Pot Roast, 81
  Roasted BBQ Turkey Drumsticks, 71
  Roasted Veggie Salad with Feta, 39
  Savory Chicken, Tomato, and
      Mushroom Stew, 31
  Seared Tuna Steaks with Slaw, 91
  Sheet Pan Breakfast Bake, 17
  Sheet Pan Sausage, Poblano
      Pepper, and Potatoes, 82
  Simple Baked Black Bean Huevos
      Rancheros, 14
  Simple Beef and Black Bean Chili, 34
  Smoked Sausage and Potato Stew, 32
  Soy-Marinated Flank Steak, 77
  Summer Arugula Salad with Watermelon, 35
  Summer Squash Marinara, 112
  Summer Squash "Pasta" with Peas, 113
  Sunday Roast Chicken Dinner, 70
  Super Easy Chicken Fried Rice, 57
  Sweet and Savory Butternut Squash Soup, 26
  30-Minute Minestrone, 27
  Tomato-Basil Gnocchi, 48
  Tortellini Soup with Italian Sausage
      and Baby Kale, 29
  Turkey Cutlets with White Wine
      and Mushrooms, 72–73
  The Ultimate Philly Cheesesteak, 80
  Wilted Balsamic Spinach, 115
  Yogurt Banana Split, 21
Onions
  French Onion Burgers, 75
  Pierogi with Fried Onions and
      Cabbage, 103
Oregano Chicken Skewers with
    Yogurt Sauce, Lemon, 66

P

Pancakes, Simple Buttermilk, 23
Pantry staples, 5
Pasta and noodles
  Black Pepper Spaghetti with
      Garlic and Parmesan, 50
  Easiest Baked Mac and Cheese, 51
  Easy Baked Ziti Casserole, 54
  Lemon Chicken Orzo Soup, 28
  Penne Florentine with Bacon, 55
  Penne with Broccoli Pesto, 52
  Rigatoni with Sausage and Chunky
      Tomato Sauce, 56
  Shrimp Orzo Skillet, 53
  Spicy Peanut Noodles, 49
  30-Minute Minestrone, 27
  Tomato-Basil Gnocchi, 48
  Tortellini Soup with Italian Sausage
      and Baby Kale, 29
Peach and Granola Crisp, 128
Peanut Noodles, Spicy, 49
Pear Bread Pudding, 123
Peas
  Garlicky Peas and Mushrooms, 116
  Summer Squash "Pasta" with Peas, 113
Peppery Chicken-Fried Cube Steaks, 79
Pesto, Penne with Broccoli, 52
Pie, Luscious Lemon, 126
Pierogi with Fried Onions and Cabbage, 103

Pineapple
  Hawaiian Pork and Pineapple Kebabs, 83
  Old-Fashioned Ambrosia, 121
Pizza, Easy Grandma Pie, 102
Poblano Pepper, and Potatoes,
    Sheet Pan Sausage, 82
Pork. *See also* Bacon; Ham; Sausage
  Hawaiian Pork and Pineapple Kebabs, 83
  Lemon Pepper Pork Tenderloin with
    Roasted Root Vegetables, 86–87
  Open-Faced Pulled Pork Sandwiches, 84
  Pork Chop Fajita Skillet, 85
Potatoes
  Garlic Roasted Potatoes with Rosemary, 109
  Ham, Bean, and Potato Soup, 30
  Sheet Pan Baked Fish and Chips, 90
  Sheet Pan Breakfast Bake, 17
  Sheet Pan Sausage, Poblano
    Pepper, and Potatoes, 82
  Smoked Sausage and Potato Stew, 32

Q

Quesadillas, Pinto Bean and Spinach, 105
Quiche, Swiss Mushroom, 99
Quick prep
  Arugula Shrimp Salad with Lemon Olive Oil, 41
  Baby Greens Salad with Beets
    and Goat Cheese, 40
  Baked Chicken Thighs with
    Tomatoes and Feta, 69
  Baked Egg and Sausage Breakfast Taquitos, 15
  Baked Oat Banana Muffins, 19
  Baked Sweet Potatoes with
    Cinnamon Honey, 108
  Black Pepper Spaghetti with
    Garlic and Parmesan, 50
  Blue Cheese and Bacon Wedge Salad, 44
  Brown Sugar Apple Galette, 127
  Buffalo Cauliflower Tacos, 106
  California Veggie Barley Bowls, 59
  Caprese Corn and Tomato Salad, 37
  Cheesy Roasted Cauliflower, 110
  Chicken and White Bean Chili, 33

Chicken Milanese with Arugula, 68
Chili Butter Corn on the Cob, 117
Chocolate-Avocado Smoothie, 22
Chopped Mediterranean Salad, 38
Couscous with Lemon Chicken and Olives, 62
Crispy Baked Carrot Fries, 111
Easiest Baked Mac and Cheese, 51
Easiest Butternut Squash Risotto, 58
Easy Baked Ziti Casserole, 54
Easy Cocoa Brownies, 125
Easy Tofu and Broccoli Stir-Fry, 96
Easy Tuna and Avocado Panzanella Salad, 42
Farro with Zucchini and Walnuts, 60–61
French Onion Burgers, 75
Garlicky Peas and Mushrooms, 116
Garlic Roasted Potatoes with Rosemary, 109
Ground Beef and String Bean Stir-Fry, 74
Ham, Bean, and Potato Soup, 30
Hawaiian Pork and Pineappled Kebabs, 83
Hearty Salmon Avocado Toast, 18
Honey-Lime Fruit Salad, 120
Lemon and Herb Scallops, 93
Lemon Chicken Orzo Soup, 28
Lemon-Dill Salmon Packet, 89
Lemon Pepper Pork Tenderloin with
    Roasted Root Vegetables, 86–87
Lentil Sloppy Joes, 98
Luscious Lemon Pie, 126
Old-Fashioned Ambrosia, 121
Open-Faced Pulled Pork Sandwiches, 84
Parmesan Baked Artichoke Hearts, 114
Parmesan Baked Asparagus and Eggs, 97
Peach and Granola Crisp, 128
Pear Bread Pudding, 123
Penne Florentine with Bacon, 55
Penne with Broccoli Pesto, 52
Peppery Chicken-Fried Cube Steaks, 79
Pierogi with Fried Onions and Cabbage, 103
Pinto Bean and Spinach Quesadillas, 105
Pork Chop Fajita Skillet, 85
Quinoa with Spicy Black Beans and
    Sausage, 63
Red Gravy Pot Roast, 81

Quick prep (*continued*)

Rigatoni with Sausage and Chunky Tomato Sauce, 56

Roasted BBQ Turkey Drumsticks, 71

Roasted Veggie Salad with Feta, 39

Savory Breakfast Egg Muffins, 16

Savory Chicken, Tomato, and Mushroom Stew, 31

Seared Tuna Steaks with Slaw, 91

Sheet Pan Breakfast Bake, 17

Sheet Pan Sausage, Poblano Pepper, and Potatoes, 82

Shrimp and Avocado Tostadas, 92

Shrimp Orzo Skillet, 53

Simple Baked Black Bean Huevos Rancheros, 14

Simple Beef and Black Bean Chili, 34

Simple Buttermilk Pancakes, 23

Smoked Sausage and Potato Stew, 32

Spicy Peanut Noodles, 49

Spinach Salad with Eggs and Bacon, 43

Strawberry Cheesecake Toast, 20

Strawberry, Spinach, and Mozzarella Salad, 36

Summer Arugula Salad with Watermelon, 35

Summer Squash Marinara, 112

Summer Squash "Pasta" with Peas, 113

Sunday Roast Chicken Dinner, 70

Super Easy Chicken Fried Rice, 57

Swiss Mushroom Quiche, 99

30-Minute Minestrone, 27

Tomato-Basil Gnocchi, 48

Tortellini Soup with Italian Sausage and Baby Kale, 29

Turkey Cutlets with White Wine and Mushrooms, 72–73

The Ultimate Philly Cheesesteak, 80

Wilted Balsamic Spinach, 115

Yogurt Banana Split, 21

Quinoa with Spicy Black Beans and Sausage, 63

R

Raspberry-Filled Butter Cookies, 124

Recipes, about, 11

Red Gravy Pot Roast, 81

Rice

Easiest Butternut Squash Risotto, 58

Super Easy Chicken Fried Rice, 57

Rosemary, Garlic Roasted Potatoes with, 109

S

Salads

Arugula Shrimp Salad with Lemon Olive Oil, 41

Baby Greens Salad with Beets and Goat Cheese, 40

Blue Cheese and Bacon Wedge Salad, 44

Caprese Corn and Tomato Salad, 37

Chopped Mediterranean Salad, 38

Easy Tuna and Avocado Panzanella Salad, 42

Honey-Lime Fruit Salad, 120

Old-Fashioned Ambrosia, 121

Roasted Veggie Salad with Feta, 39

Spinach Salad with Eggs and Bacon, 43

Strawberry, Spinach, and Mozzarella Salad, 36

Summer Arugula Salad with Watermelon, 35

Salmon

Hearty Salmon Avocado Toast, 18

Lemon-Dill Salmon Packet, 89

Sheet Pan Lemon-Garlic Salmon and Veggie Bowl, 88

Salsa

Chicken Enchiladas Verde, 67

Simple Baked Black Bean Huevos Rancheros, 14

Sandwiches. *See also* Burgers; Toast

Lentil Sloppy Joes, 98

Open-Faced Pulled Pork Sandwiches, 84

The Ultimate Philly Cheesesteak, 80

Sausage

Baked Egg and Sausage Breakfast Taquitos, 15

Quinoa with Spicy Black Beans and Sausage, 63

Rigatoni with Sausage and Chunky Tomato Sauce, 56

Sheet Pan Sausage, Poblano Pepper, and Potatoes, 82

Smoked Sausage and Potato Stew, 32

Tortellini Soup with Italian Sausage and Baby Kale, 29

Scallops, Lemon and Herb, 93

Shrimp
  Arugula Shrimp Salad with Lemon Olive Oil, 41
  Shrimp and Avocado Tostadas, 92
  Shrimp Orzo Skillet, 53
Slaw, Seared Tuna Steaks with, 91
Smoothie, Chocolate Avocado, 22
Soups, stews, and chilis
  Chicken and White Bean Chili, 33
  Ham, Bean, and Potato Soup, 30
  Lemon Chicken Orzo Soup, 28
  Savory Chicken, Tomato, and
    Mushroom Stew, 31
  Simple Beef and Black Bean Chili, 34
  Smoked Sausage and Potato Stew, 32
  Sweet and Savory Butternut Squash Soup, 26
  30-Minute Minestrone, 27
  Tortellini Soup with Italian Sausage
    and Baby Kale, 29
Soy-Marinated Flank Steak, 77
Spinach
  Penne Florentine with Bacon, 55
  Pinto Bean and Spinach Quesadillas, 105
  Spinach Salad with Eggs and Bacon, 43
  Strawberry, Spinach, and Mozzarella
    Salad, 36
  Wilted Balsamic Spinach, 115
Squash
  Easiest Butternut Squash Risotto, 58
  Summer Squash Marinara, 112
  Summer Squash "Pasta" with Peas, 113
  Sweet and Savory Butternut Squash Soup, 26
Stir-fries
  Easy Tofu and Broccoli Stir-Fry, 96
  Ground Beef and String Bean Stir-Fry, 74
Strawberries
  Chocolate-Dipped Strawberries, 122
  Strawberry Cheesecake Toast, 20
  Strawberry, Spinach, and Mozzarella Salad, 36
String Bean Stir-Fry, Ground Beef and, 74
Substitutions, 4
Summer Arugula Salad with Watermelon, 35
Sweet Potatoes with Cinnamon Honey, Baked, 108

T
Tacos, Buffalo Cauliflower, 106
30 minutes or less
  Arugula Shrimp Salad with Lemon
    Olive Oil, 41
  Baby Greens Salad with Beets
    and Goat Cheese, 40
  Baked Oat Banana Muffins, 19
  Black Pepper Spaghetti with
    Garlic and Parmesan, 50
  Blue Cheese and Bacon Wedge Salad, 44
  Brown Sugar Apple Galette, 127
  Buffalo Cauliflower Tacos, 106
  Chili Butter Corn on the Cob, 117
  Chocolate-Avocado Smoothie, 22
  Chopped Mediterranean Salad, 38
  Couscous with Lemon Chicken and Olives, 62
  Crispy Baked Carrot Fries, 111
  Easy Tuna and Avocado Panzanella Salad, 42
  Garlicky Peas and Mushrooms, 116
  Ground Beef and String Bean Stir-Fry, 74
  Hearty Salmon Avocado Toast, 18
  Honey-Lime Fruit Salad, 120
  Lemon and Herb Scallops, 93
  Lemon Chicken Orzo Soup, 28
  Lemon-Dill Salmon Packet, 89
  Old-Fashioned Ambrosia, 121
  Parmesan Baked Artichoke Hearts, 114
  Parmesan Baked Asparagus and Eggs, 97
  Penne with Broccoli Pesto, 52
  Pierogi with Fried Onions and Cabbage, 103
  Pinto Bean and Spinach Quesadillas, 105
  Roasted Veggie Salad with Feta, 39
  Seared Tuna Steaks with Slaw, 91
  Shrimp and Avocado Tostadas, 92
  Simple Buttermilk Pancakes, 23
  Spicy Peanut Noodles, 49
  Spinach Salad with Eggs and Bacon, 43
  Strawberry Cheesecake Toast, 20
  Strawberry, Spinach, and Mozzarella Salad, 36
  Summer Arugula Salad with Watermelon, 35
  Summer Squash Marinara, 112

30 minutes or less (*continued*)
 Summer Squash "Pasta" with
  Peas, 113
 Super Easy Chicken Fried Rice, 57
 30-Minute Minestrone, 27
 Tomato-Basil Gnocchi, 48
 Tortellini Soup with Italian Sausage
  and Baby Kale, 29
 Turkey Cutlets with White Wine
  and Mushrooms, 72–73
 Wilted Balsamic Spinach, 115
 Yogurt Banana Split, 21
Toast
 Hearty Salmon Avocado Toast, 18
 Strawberry Cheesecake Toast, 20
Tofu
 Baked BBQ Tofu and Broccoli, 104
 Easy Tofu and Broccoli Stir-Fry, 96
Tomatoes
 Baked Chicken Thighs with
  Tomatoes and Feta, 69
 Caprese Corn and Tomato Salad, 37
 Rigatoni with Sausage and Chunky
  Tomato Sauce, 56
 Savory Chicken, Tomato, and
  Mushroom Stew, 31
 Summer Squash Marinara, 112
 30-Minute Minestrone, 27
 Tomato-Basil Gnocchi, 48
Tortillas
 Baked Egg and Sausage Breakfast
  Taquitos, 15
 Chicken Enchiladas Verde, 67
 Pinto Bean and Spinach Quesadillas, 105
 Shrimp and Avocado Tostadas, 92
Tuna
 Easy Tuna and Avocado Panzanella
  Salad, 42
 Seared Tuna Steaks with Slaw, 91
Turkey
 Roasted BBQ Turkey Drumsticks, 71
 Turkey Cutlets with White Wine
  and Mushrooms, 72–73

V
Vegan
 Baked BBQ Tofu and Broccoli, 104
 The Best Black Bean Burgers, 100–101
 California Veggie Barley Bowls, 59
 Crispy Baked Carrot Fries, 111
 Garlicky Peas and Mushrooms, 116
 Garlic Roasted Potatoes with Rosemary, 109
 Lentil Sloppy Joes, 98
 Spicy Peanut Noodles, 49
 30-Minute Minestrone, 27
 Wilted Balsamic Spinach, 115
Vegetables. *See also specific*
 California Veggie Barley Bowls, 59
 Lemon Pepper Pork Tenderloin with
  Roasted Root Vegetables, 86–87
 Roasted Veggie Salad with Feta, 39
 Sheet Pan Lemon-Garlic Salmon
  and Veggie Bowl, 88
 Super Easy Chicken Fried Rice, 57
 30-Minute Minestrone, 27
Vegetarian. *See also Vegan*
 Baby Greens Salad with Beets
  and Goat Cheese, 40
 Baked Oat Banana Muffins, 19
 Baked Sweet Potatoes with
  Cinnamon Honey, 108
 Black Pepper Spaghetti with
  Garlic and Parmesan, 50
 Brown Sugar Apple Galette, 127
 Buffalo Cauliflower Tacos, 106
 Caprese Corn and Tomato Salad, 37
 Cheesy Roasted Cauliflower, 110
 Chili Butter Corn on the Cob, 117
 Chocolate-Avocado Smoothie, 22
 Chocolate-Dipped Strawberries, 122
 Chopped Mediterranean Salad, 38
 Easiest Baked Mac and Cheese, 51
 Easiest Butternut Squash Risotto, 58
 Easy Cocoa Brownies, 125
 Easy Grandma Pie Pizza, 102
 Easy Tofu and Broccoli Stir-Fry, 96

Farro with Zucchini and Walnuts, 60–61

Honey-Lime Fruit Salad, 120

Lasagna-Stuffed Zucchini Boats, 107

Luscious Lemon Pie, 126

Parmesan Baked Artichoke Hearts, 114

Parmesan Baked Asparagus and Eggs, 97

Peach and Granola Crisp, 128

Pear Bread Pudding, 123

Penne with Broccoli Pesto, 52

Pierogi with Fried Onions and Cabbage, 103

Pinto Bean and Spinach Quesadillas, 105

Raspberry-Filled Butter Cookies, 124

Roasted Veggie Salad with Feta, 39

Simple Baked Black Bean Huevos Rancheros, 14

Simple Buttermilk Pancakes, 23

Strawberry Cheesecake Toast, 20

Strawberry, Spinach, and Mozzarella Salad, 36

Summer Arugula Salad with Watermelon, 35

Summer Squash Marinara, 112

Summer Squash "Pasta" with Peas, 113

Sweet and Savory Butternut Squash Soup, 26

Swiss Mushroom Quiche, 99

Tomato-Basil Gnocchi, 48

Yogurt Banana Split, 21

W

Walnuts, Farro with Zucchini and, 60–61

Watermelon, Summer Arugula Salad with, 35

White Wine and Mushrooms, Turkey Cutlets with, 72–73

Whole foods, 4–5

Y

Yogurt
  Lemon Oregano Chicken Skewers with Yogurt Sauce, 66
  Strawberry Cheesecake Toast, 20
  Yogurt Banana Split, 21

Z

Zucchini
  Farro with Zucchini and Walnuts, 60–61
  Lasagna-Stuffed Zucchini Boats, 107
  Summer Squash Marinara, 112
  Summer Squash "Pasta" with Peas, 113

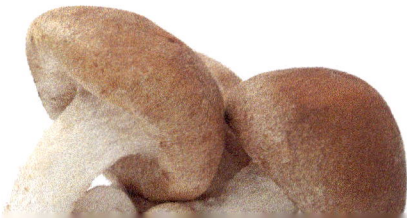

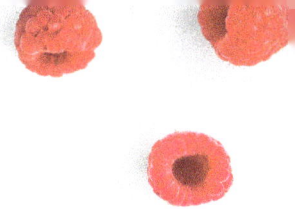

Acknowledgments

It has been an absolute dream to author a family-based cookbook. I am beyond grateful for the numerous mentors and colleagues who have offered continual support throughout my career. To all of my registered dietitian nutritionist colleagues who have provided inspiration, motivation, and encouragement over the past two decades, so many of you have helped show me a path and inspired me to push a little harder each and every day. You have shown me you can do whatever you put your mind to!

This book could have not been written without the support of my husband, parents, and kiddos. My husband is my rock and support and is always (well, almost always) willing to try my recipe creations. Thanks to my parents and in-laws, who have always supported and encouraged me regardless of my next venture or project idea (and, trust me, there have been a lot over the past few decades), and to my kiddos for their gracious love and willingness to allow me to spend some extra time in the kitchen as I prepared this book.

And of course, a big thank-you to the team at Callisto Media for having confidence in me to develop this project and for making this whole process extremely smooth. Thank you!

About the Author

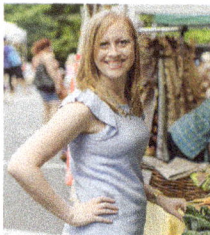

Kristen Smith, MS, RDN, is a registered dietitian nutritionist and the blogger behind 360FamilyNutrition.org. She is the mother of two young boys and truly understands the challenges behind feeding a family. Kristen has worked in the field of nutrition for the past two decades, specializing in family nutrition and weight management. She is currently a spokesperson for the Academy of Nutrition and Dietetics and has been quoted in hundreds of media interviews. Kristen's nutrition expertise has been featured on *Good Morning America* and in *The New York Times, U.S. News & World Report*, and many more outlets. In her spare time Kristen loves to travel, spend time outdoors with her family, and create festive snack boards.

About the Recipe Developer

Lisa Grant is the author of several cookbooks and the blogger behind JerseyGirlCooks.com. She is married and has two almost-grown children. While she loves to travel, her favorite place is her kitchen in New Jersey. Lisa's Italian/Croatian heritage shines in her cooking. Her passion is to spread her love of food to others by sharing her easy recipes and simple cooking tips.

www.ingramcontent.com/pod-product-compliance
Lightning Source LLC
Chambersburg PA
CBHW051258110426
42743CB00054B/3485